The Miracle
of
Metaphysical Healing

Evelyn M. Monahan

Parker Publishing Company, Inc.
West Nyack, New York

© 1975, *by*

PARKER PUBLISHING COMPANY, INC.

West Nyack, N.Y.

Reward Edition . . . . . June 1977

Fourth Printing . . . . . March, 1980

This book is a reference work based on research by
the author. The opinions expressed herein are not
necessarily those of or endorsed by the Publisher.

Library of Congress Cataloging in Publication Data

Monahan, Evelyn.
    The miracle of metaphysical healing.

    1. Mental healing. I. Title.
RZ401.M74   615'.851   75-12721

Printed in the United States of America

To my best friend:
Betty C. Reaid,
who touched my life with the miracle
of metaphysical healing

How Metaphysical Healing Can Bring You A Wonderful New Life

Have you ever suffered the agonizing pain of illness or injury? Have you ever stood by helplessly and watched someone you love tortured by the pain of an unwanted illness? Have you ever spent a sleepless night after discovering that a friend or loved one is suffering from a disease which doctors have pronounced incurable? Do you know a person in your own family or in the family of a friend who has become a slave to drugs or alcohol? Are there family ties or friendships in your life which have been torn apart by bitterness and resentments? Does the lack of money add new pain to your everyday life? Is there anything about your physical or emotional health which you would like to change? Is there any situation in your life which you consider in need of healing?

If your answer to any one of these questions is yes, then this book is written especially for you. In this book you will learn the secrets of metaphysical healing which will bring new health to your body, your mind, and every area of your life.

With the very first chapter of this book you will find that your attitude toward living takes on a new and healthy outlook. You will discover your own power to live your life free of pain, illness, and worry. Each additional chapter will place in your hands a new key which will unlock doors previously closed to you. Each page of this book is a map which will lead you to your own power to control not only your physical health, but your entire life.

There are no complicated techniques to follow in order to use these secrets to your own advantage. You will have no trouble understanding the methods by which you may begin to use this power today. Metaphysical healing is the strongest force in the entire universe, and you can begin to use this force within the next 15 minutes.

There are many books available today which talk about positive thinking, but not one of these books deals with the power which will be placed in your hands in the following chapters of this book. That force is the power of metaphysical healing made possible through the secrets of energized mind. You will learn to use your mind as an all-powerful force in creating new health for yourself and for those you love, and you will learn to do this not next month or next week, but today!

I have made the techniques very simple to follow—don't let the simplicity fool you. A stick of dynamite can look like a very simple object and, yet, the force it can unleash can move mountains. These techniques of metaphysical healing contain the dynamite to move any mountains which are obstructing your health or your attainment of any desired goal! Few people throughout history have been fortunate enough to learn these techniques since they were usually presented cloaked in a veil of mystery. I have removed that veil for you and placed at your fingertips the means by which you can live the rest of your life free of pain and illness and free from the lack of any goal you desire.

I have used these techniques myself and I have found their effects astounding! Twelve years ago, I was involved in an accident which left me blind. Since my blindness was a result of a head injury, all the doctors who examined me stated that my blindness was a permanent condition and could never be healed through any means known to medicine. At the age of 22 years, I was faced with the prospect of living the rest of my life in a world of darkness.

The same head injury which had claimed my eyesight also left me with epilepsy. I experienced as many as 12 epileptic seizures a day and was placed on medication in an attempt to control these seizures. Despite the daily use of medications, I still experienced as many as ten epileptic seizures a day. At this point, with my eyesight gone, and with the additional handicap of epileptic seizures, my future looked anything but bright. If anyone had told me at that time that things could be worse, I doubt that I would have believed them.

Four years later things did get worse. I was involved in an accident which left my right arm paralyzed. Since I am naturally right-handed, this meant an additional burden in my already bleak existence. If the future looked bleak to me before, it now looked completely black. I had always been an independent person and I found my necessary dependence upon others extremely frustrating. In spite of the fact that friends gladly offered their help, I was angry with myself and with life for placing me in a position where I could not be a completely independent individual.

After nine years of feeling sorry for myself and allowing bitterness and resentment to replace my better judgment, I decided to do something about my situation. I had long since accepted the fact that medicine could offer nothing to help my blindness, my epilepsy, or my paralyzed right arm. I began to think seriously concerning the idea of metaphysical healing. Since childhood, I had heard stories of people who had received miraculous healings when doctors and medicine could offer them no hope. I had always been interested in the field of the occult. I began to recall some of the things I had learned as a child. I had absolutely nothing to lose and everything to gain.

After thinking for many days on all the information that had come into my life since my childhood concerning metaphysical healing, I decided to take the steps necessary to effect my own complete cure from blindness, epilepsy, and paralysis. I shared my ideas with two close friends and asked them if they would aid me in the metaphysical healing techniques which I felt would bring about my complete cure. They agreed to follow my directions and the three of us began immediately to put into practice the secrets I had discovered.

Ten days after beginning to use the techniques of metaphysical healing, my eyesight returned to me, instantaneously. At this time, I noticed that I was not experiencing any epileptic seizures. After consulting my physician concerning my epilepsy and explaining to him the fact that I felt I had been cured, he agreed to run several tests. The tests revealed that I had no more evidence of epilepsy. It was no longer necessary for me to take the daily medication which had been an important part of my life for nine long years. I have not experienced an epileptic seizure since that fateful day when my eyesight was returned to me.

One week after the return of my eyesight, my right arm was freed from the paralysis which had held it immobile for several long years. I was able to move my arm freely, and the pain which had been my constant companion over the long years of paralysis had disappeared. I had so much for which to be thankful, and a lot to think

about. I had found secrets of metaphysical healing and I was determined to make the secrets available to every man, woman, and child
on this planet.

I had managed, in spite of my handicaps, to complete my
undergraduate work at the University of Tennessee where I received
a bachelors degree in Psychology and Sociology. I had accomplished
this with the aid of recorded textbooks and the help of friends who
would read my assignments to me aloud. In this same manner, I had
been able to complete a year of graduate work in experimental
psychology at Emory University in Atlanta. I decided to return to
school to work toward my Ph.D. in Educational Psychology at
Georgia State University in Atlanta. I also decided that I would teach
Parapsychology at Georgia State University. The fact that such a
course had never been taught at this university or at any other
university did not discourage me at this point. I felt that if metaphysical healing could be used to such an extent as to bring about the cures
it had worked for me, that it could also be used to heal any situation in
my life. I began to use these same secrets that had brought about my
healing toward the goal of teaching classes at Georgia State University and making these same secrets available to my students.

I telephoned the University and explained to a secretary exactly
what I wanted to do. The secretary politely took my name and
telephone number and said that if anyone at the University was
interested, she would contact me at a later date. One month went by
and I had not heard a word from the University. Then, one morning
my telephone rang and I was asked by the Director of Special Studies
at Georgia State University if I would still like to teach a class in
Parapsychology. I was to speak to him that very afternoon and since I
had enough confidence in the secrets of metaphysical healing, I had
already prepared the curriculum for such a course. During our meeting, I explained to this gentleman my ideas for teaching the course
and presented him with a copy of the curriculum I had outlined. My
educational qualifications were checked and I was offered the position of Instructor of Parapsychology at Georgia State University
School of Special Studies in Atlanta, Georgia. My classes have
drawn on an average of 250 students per quarter.

I realized that if I were to make the secrets of energized mind
available to the number of people who could benefit from them, it
was necessary for me to receive the aid of radio, television, newspa-
pers, and magazines. With this goal in mind, I began to use the

secrets again in order to heal whatever situation stood in my way of receiving space in such publications and air time on broadcasting networks. One month after I began teaching classes, the *Atlanta Journal* contacted me and asked to do a story regarding the classes which I taught. The following week, I was contacted by WSB Television and asked to appear on "Today In Georgia," a program broadcasted throughout the state, reaching millions of viewers. Audience response to my appearance on this program was so great that three weeks later I was asked to return and, this time, I was given twice the air time I was allowed on the first program. The techniques of metaphysical healing worked so well that I was bombarded by requests to appear on local radio and TV stations throughout the state of Georgia. *Atlanta Magazine* devoted its profile story for the month of August, 1972, to me and my classes at Georgia State University. The opportunity of reaching people on a national level was also afforded to me through the techniques of metaphysical healing. *Newsweek* did a story in their Educational Section on me and my classes in their issue published August 28, 1972. This was followed by requests to appear on national TV programs and write-ups in other national publications, such as the *National Inquirer*, *Midnight*, and *Time* Magazine. Five different publishing houses have asked me to submit manuscripts to their companies for publication. My first book is in the process of being published in Japan, England, Germany, Mexico, and Italy. Through the power of metaphysical healing I am constantly being presented with the opportunity of reaching increasingly larger numbers of people.

With the techniques I have outlined for you in this book, I have been able to change my entire life, stepping away from the prospect of living my life in total darkness, experiencing daily epileptic seizures, and knowing the restrictions of paralysis. I have taught these techniques to my students and I now wish to teach them to you. This book is my means of contacting you, personally. With each page you read, I will involve you more and more in the use of metaphysical healing, so that you may change any situation in your life which is in need of healing. You will learn not only how to heal your physical body and your mind, but, also, how to heal economic situations, family ties, broken friendships, and how to turn bleak prospects into bright promises. Notice that I have not said you *can* learn this, but you *will* learn this. The further you read in this book, the more will the secrets of metaphysical healing penetrate into every area of your life. There is no way you can avoid the use of these secrets if you have read this book. Your higher mind will grasp ideas and techniques without your even realizing that they have been taken into your everyday life. You will be astounded to realize that the things you only wished were possible for you, have, actually, materialized in your life through the power of energized mind.

I have seen countless numbers of people use these techniques to bring about healing of their body, mind, and life situations, and in the following chapters, I will share with you the story of some of these people. They have given their permission for their stories to be told in order that you may realize that no special I.Q. requirements are needed, no special financial status, and no special formal education is needed in order to put these secrets to work in order to completely change your life.

Begin now, and read the first chapter of this book. Remember as you read, that I am speaking especially to you. In spite of the fact that a million other people may read this book, it is written for you, personally. Each chapter will tell *you* how to use metaphysical healing immediately. Chapter two will tell you how to use metaphysical healing in order to heal your financial life. In Chapter three, you will discover the secrets of using metaphysical healing to help those you love. Each chapter will bring you additional secrets that will work for you, personally.

Begin immediately to read this book, so that you need not spend one more hour without the secret of metaphysical healing in your life. Join, now, with the increasing number of fortunate people who have discovered the secrets of energized mind.

Evelyn M. Monahan

Contents

The Miracle
of
Metaphysical Healing

one

You Can Use the Miracle of Metaphysical Healing to Work Wonders

The miracle power of metaphysical healing is within you this very minute. Since the first moment of your birth you have had the miracle power to heal. If you have not used your ability to heal thus far in your life, you have already lived too long without the benefits it can bring to your mind and body.

The key to the miracle of metaphysical healing lies within a special area and quality of your own mind. In the following pages of this book you will learn how to reach the special area of the mind and use the special quality of the mind which brings cures from all illness and injuries. This special area of your mind is called your higher self, and the special quality it possesses is called ENERGIZED MIND.

THE HIGHER MIND AND HOW TO REACH IT

Your mind is like a house with many rooms. Just as the rooms of a house are designated for a special purpose, the rooms or areas of your mind also have a special purpose which is theirs and theirs alone. Most men spend their life in an area known as conscious mind. In this area of mind is stored all your fears, all your self-imposed limitations, and all words such as incurable, cannot, impossible, and no hope. Conscious mind has little or no confidence in itself and is far too anxious to listen to and believe all limitations placed upon you since your childhood. It is a passive area of your being that is blind to the reality of a higher self which knows no limitations and is capable of achieving anything. Sickness and disease of all kinds have made their way into men's bodies through this inert area of man's thinking. Energized mind cuts through the false thinking of conscious mind as easily as a laser beam cuts through butter.

Energized mind exists within the high self. This special area of your mind knows the truth about you. The high self knows that incurable, cannot, and no hope are only words and have no real meaning in your life. The high self does not need confidence, for it is itself confidence since it knows well its own limitless power. The high self is constantly aware of the fact that it is in total control of your physical body and can destroy any illness or injury which would cause the body pain or suffering. It is an area of yourself that is always on your side. It stands ready to maintain perfect health in your mind and body and to restore that health if it is ever lost through the false beliefs of conscious mind.

Far from being passive, the high self has a limitless store of energy. In order for you to have this limitless energy at your disposal, it is necessary only that you make contact with your higher self. Once this contact has been made, sickness, injury, pain, and suffering will be only dim memories in your past, for you will have reached the key to the miracle of metaphysical healing. The technique that follows is a failproof method of reaching the higher mind in yourself. Begin now and practice this technique at least three times a day. It is the first step in bringing the miracle of healing to your own mind and body

YOUR TECHNIQUE FOR REACHING YOUR HIGHER SELF

1. Choose a quiet place where you are not likely to be interrupted. Sit in a comfortable chair whose back is high enough to support your head. (If it is possible to lie down, this is an excellent position for beginning this technique.)

2. Sit without crossing your arms or legs, and close your eyes. Take a deep breath through your nose and visualize or imagine that breath flowing through your entire body and coming back to rest in your head. Repeat this breathing technique three times, allowing yourself to be aware that energy is in the breath and will follow your visualization through this exercise.

3. Repeat the following words to yourself: "I am a magnificent numan being. I am without equal in all of creation. My mind and

body are so magnificently constructed that no feat of engineering could ever duplicate the uniqueness in myself. I will transcend all ordinary thinking and dwell entirely in my higher self.''

4. Take a deep breath through your nose and visualize the breath circulating through your body and again coming to rest within the center of your brain. Repeat this exercise three times.

5. Repeat the following words three times: ''In the awareness of my higher self, I know no limits. My will is the strongest force in all of creation. I will now to be in ever-increasing contact with my higher self.''

This technique will allow you to reach and maintain contact with your high self throughout your life. That contact will put at your disposal all the power of energized mind. With that power and the techniques that follow in this book you will be able to rid yourself, your loved ones, and all situations in your life from the immobilizing grip of pain, sickness, and disease. You will be able to bring health to all areas of your life—physical, mental, emotional, or economic —which have been ravaged by pain or sorrow, for the miracle of metaphysical healing knows no limits to its possibilities.

Since you live in a world where your conscious mind is constantly bombarded by ads and commercials selling sickness and poor health to a gullible public, the area of physical health will be of prime interest to you in using the miracle power of metaphysical healing.

METAPHYSICAL HEALING BRINGS FREEDOM FROM ARTHRITIS

Countless numbers of people have had their health restored to them through the miracle of metaphysical healing. Robert W. is one such person.

I met Robert a little over one year ago, and it was obvious before Robert spoke that he was suffering severe pain from the crippling effects of arthritis. The fingers of both hands were swollen and restricted in movement. He had the gait of an old man despite the fact that he was only 37 years old. As Robert talked with me, the state of his body and mind, severely battered by arthritis, unfolded itself in a story of years of pain and suffering.

"I've had this condition for four years and nothing I do brings any relief," he said while looking directly into my eyes. "I've heard about your healing and I want to know if the same thing can happen for me?"

He seemed almost afraid that my answer would be "No" and despite the fact that he was in severe physical pain relief showed on his face as I responded to his question. "I'm not special, Robert. You are capable of bringing healing to yourself just as I brought healing to myself. If you are serious about wanting to be cured all you need do is follow the laws and techniques for metaphysical healing."

We talked for an hour and a half, and Robert assured me that he wanted more than anything in the world to be free of the pain of arthritis which had twisted his hands and legs and brought pain and suffering into every moment of his life. Robert agreed to follow the techniques which I outlined for him and to get back in touch with me within two weeks. He made it clear that he would have to use the telephone since his arthritic condition made it impossible for him to write with a pen or pencil or to even use a typewriter. We parted company and Robert left with a sheet of paper I had given to him which contained the method for bringing about the miracle of metaphysical healing.

Two weeks passed and I had not heard from Robert W. I was delighted when three days after the appointed time when Robert was supposed to contact me I opened a letter to find that it had been written by Robert by hand. The letter stated that the effects of metaphysical healing became apparent so quickly that he had decided to wait until he was able to use a pen in order to announce to me his cure and also to express his thanks for sharing with him this miracle method for healing. He went on to say that I was receiving the first letter he had been able to write in one and a half years since this was the first time in that period that his fingers had allowed him freedom of movement and freedom from pain so that he might use a pen freely to express his thoughts. The letter bubbled with excitement and a P.S. brought an extra bonus smile to my face. That P.S. was to tell me that Robert had walked two blocks in order to place his letter in the mailbox himself.

Although I was very happy that Robert had found freedom from arthritis, I was not in the least bit surprised. I still hear from Robert every once in a while and he is pursuing his profession as a top-flight automobile mechanic.

THE IMPORTANCE OF REJECTING NEGATIVE THINKING

One fact which all people who have received their health through the miracle of metaphysical healing have in common is the rejection of negative thinking. The conscious mind is very good at accepting all suggestion that comes into it. If it believes the body which it inhabits is sick with disease or tortured by pain, that body will suffer the consequences of those thoughts. The power to reason is a wonderful gift to all human beings, but there is a force that lies without the reasoning ability of all all human beings by virtue of the fact that it taps the infinite. The higher self is man's road to tapping that infinite source of power and it will bring into actualization any thought which the conscious mind believes. If a man clutters his thinking with negative thoughts he can expect his life to be cluttered with negative and unhealthy circumstances.

It is unfortunate that the world in which you live is inhabited by so many people who allow negative thinking to rule their life. More sad still is the fact that many of these people would impose their negative thinking upon you and your family. A very bright spot in all of this is the fact that you have the ability to reject all negative thought. In truth, negative thinking is itself a disease which brings pain, suffering, and even death into the lives of those who allow it to rule their lives. You need never let this happen to you. Your first step in combating negative thinking is never to allow yourself to dwell on a negative thought. In Chapter ten of this book you will learn how to deal effectively with all negative thoughts, whether those thoughts come to you from other people or have their beginnings within your own conscious mind. The secret to keep uppermost in your mind right now is NEVER ALLOW YOURSELF TO DWELL ON NEGATIVE THOUGHTS!

NEGATIVE THINKING KEPT A MAN IN PAIN FOR FOUR LONG YEARS

When I first met Roy M. he was wearing a back brace and was unable to take part in any strenuous physical activity. His first statement to me was filled with negative thinking: "You do a lot of talking about this miracle healing, but I know it won't work for me."

Roy looked completely shocked when I answered, "With that

kind of attitude, Mr. M., I'd be surprised if anything would work for you. Your negative thinking is keeping you a prisoner in that brace.''

We talked for approximately one hour, and Roy's conversation for the first 15 minutes was rich in negative statements. When I explained to him that his negative thoughts were one of the main reasons he was still experiencing pain in his back, he looked at me with open disbelief. I offered him a challenge. He was to stop dwelling on all negative thoughts, and start using the methods which would allow the miracle of energized mind to bring metaphysical healing to his body and his conscious mind. He agreed that he had little to lose and much to gain if just by chance what I was saying were true.

I gave Roy a step-by-step technique for using a mental paintbrush to bring the miracle of metaphysical healing to his pain-racked body and mind. Roy used the technique faithfully, and it was two weeks later when I received a phone call from him informing me that he had taken off his brace and placed it in the storeroom with some other old junk that was of no further use. He had been completely pain-free for four days and was able to move about freely with no limitations. Roy was anxious to get off the telephone since he had some work in the yard which had been waiting for him for a number of years. He stated that he would call me again in a week or so and let me know how he was progressing. Eight months and many phone calls later Roy was still without back pain and living his life without the brace he had carried around with him for four long years. He had returned to his old job as foreman in a warehouse where heavy lifting was required of him at least two or three times a day.

The last time I heard from Roy he was enthusiastically selling the idea of the miracle of energized mind to me! ''Everybody should know about the miracle of energized mind. When I think of all the time I spent in pain and wearing that brace I could kick myself for my stupidity. Instead of kicking myself though, I'm going to do everything I can to let other people know about the miracle power they have to heal their own bodies. Don't you stop telling people about this miracle of metaphysical healing. It would be criminal to keep something like that to yourself.''

Roy need not have worried since I fully intend to share the techniques of energized mind with all people who will listen and take advantage of those techniques. You can begin to take advantage of those techniques right now. The techniques which worked for Roy

M. follow on the next couple of pages. They are yours to use and will put you on your way to perfect health.

Read the technique through carefully at least two times. Then settle back and follow the step by step instructions that will lead you to a life free of illness, pain, and disease.

HOW TO PAINT YOURSELF THE PICTURE OF HEALTH THROUGH THE MIRACLE OF ENERGIZED MIND

1. Choose a place where you are not likely to be disturbed. Make yourself comfortable by lying down or sitting in a chair with a back high enough to support your head. Now you are ready to use the miracle of your mental paintbrush.

2. Close your eyes and take a deep breath through your nose. Relax your stomach muscles as soon as you have inhaled. In your mind's eye watch the breath flow throughout your entire body, ending its journey in the area of your head. Repeat this breathing technique three times.

3. Begin to use the miracle of your mental paintbrush by using your mind's eye to picture the muscles of your body. Use your mental paintbrush, allowing it to sweep across your mind and relax all your muscles beginning with your head and face and continuing through your body to your toes. In your own mind repeat the words, "I will my muscles to relax completely. I will that all unnecessary tension and stress leave my muscles now."

4. With the miracle of energized mind paint a picture in your mind's eye of your circulatory system. Allow yourself to picture all the blood vessels, arteries, and capillaries, the smaller veins throughout your entire body. As you relax even more deeply be aware of the flow of blood through your physical body. Mentally repeat the following words to yourself: "I will that my circulatory system be in perfect harmony within itself. I will that it carry all impurities out of my body, and bring new life and vitality to all the cells of my body. I will that my circulatory system be in complete harmony with all other systems of my body."

5. Paint a picture of your respiratory system in your mind's eye, using the miracle of your mental paintbrush. Allow a clear picture of your lungs to form on the screen of your inner

consciousness. With a stroke of your mental paintbrush allow motion to be added to your portrait, and watch the lungs as they expand to take in air and contract to expel impurities from your body. Mentally repeat the following words in your own mind: "I will that my respiratory system be in perfect balance within itself. I will that it shall take in oxygen and use it efficiently for my highest good. With the power of energized mind I command that my respiratory system carry cleansing oxygen to every area of my body, and carry all impurities away from the cells of my body and outside my own system. I will that my respiratory system be in complete harmony with all other systems of my body."

6. You are now ready to paint a mental picture of your digestive system. With the aid of energized mind and your mental paintbrush, form a clear picture of your stomach, small intestines, and large intestines. Repeat the following words to yourself mentally: "Through the miracle power of energized mind I will that my digestive system be in complete harmony within itself. I will that it obtain the maximum good from all food introduced into my body. With the miracle force of energized mind I command that my digestive system be in complete harmony with all other systems of my body."

7. Paint a picture in your mind of your heart. With the miracle of energized mind allow your paintbrush to add motion to the picture you have formed. Repeat the following words to yourself mentally: "With the miracle power of energized mind I command that my heart be in complete harmony within itself. I command that it work at a level of top efficiency, neither overworking nor underworking. I command that my heart be in complete harmony with all other systems of my body."

8. In the inner consciousness of your mind's eye paint a picture of your skeletal system. Allow your mental paintbrush backed by the power of energized mind to give a clear picture of all the bones and joints in your body. Repeat the following words mentally to yourself: "Through the miracle of energized mind I command that all the bones and joints of my body be in complete harmony within themselves. I command that all unnecessary calcium deposits in my joints and anywhere else in my skeletal system be dissolved and carried away from me as impurities not

in harmony with my perfect health. I will that all my joints work at their utmost level and that the skeleton of my body be in complete harmony with all other systems of my body.''

9. Now paint a picture of yourself as you would look in a photograph or painting reflecting the picture of perfect health. With this picture in your mind's eye repeat the following words to yourself mentally: ''I will that all systems of my body and mind be in complete harmony inside themselves and in relation to each other. With the miracle power of energized mind I command that my high self maintain this balance by directing all the cells of my body which are created new every day to restore or replace any cell which is diseased or injured. Through this miracle process my body shall be kept in a state of perfect health where any illness or injury will be unable to flourish and will be carried away from me as an impurity contaminating a harmonious working system.''

10. Allow yourself to be aware of all the pictures painted by you the mental artist. Be aware of the relaxation and new energy which flows throughout your entire body and mind. Take a deep breath through your nose and allow your mind to follow that breath throughout your entire body. Repeat this breathing technique three times. The following words should be repeated to yourself mentally: ''I am in perfect health in body and mind. Through the miracle of metaphysical healing and the power of energized mind I am and shall continue to be a perfectly healthy human being.'' Open your eyes and go about your daily business.

This miracle technique practiced properly will take approximately 15 minutes of your time each day. In return you will receive the blessings of perfect health in body and mind. You have been born with the miracle power to bring metaphysical healing to yourself and others. In this book you have all the techniques necessary to tap the miracle of energized mind which lies within you. You have begun your journey on the road to perfect health and in the following pages of this book you will learn all the techniques necessary to deal with any circumstance of illness, injury, or everyday life that would threaten you with pain or suffering. Learn these techniques and practice them daily; they are your means for claiming your birthright—the gift of perfect health.

two

Bring the Miracle
of Metaphysical Healing
to Those You Love

Have you ever stood by feeling helpless and watched a friend or relative suffer pain or waste away due to disease or injury? Through the miracle of metaphysical healing you are never powerless to help your loved ones regain their health. The miracle techniques contained in this book will allow you to be the motivating force in bringing health and well-being to anyone you choose to help. You will never again be placed in the situation where your only statement can be, "If only I could do something to help. If only I could help ease the pain and cure him from this illness." You are a born healer, and the techniques of metaphysical healing which will work for you without fail will also enable you to bring the miracle of healing to all of your loved ones.

You need not worry if your circle of friends and loved ones is large, for the power of energized mind which brings the miracle of metaphysical healing can never be exhausted. You will find that the more you use these miraculous techniques, the stronger will be your ability to tap this miracle force.

THE FEELING OF HELPLESSNESS BRINGS PAIN

You are well-aware that pain and sickness strikes down not only the particular victim, but spreads the disease to all those who feel love and concern for that victim. This fact has been made clear to me time and time again, but never quite so clear as it was the first quarter I taught at Emory University School of Nursing in Atlanta, Georgia.

24

In teaching senior nursing students I was constantly made aware of the terrible mental devastation suffered by the family and friends of each patient ravaged by serious pain, illness, or injury. The mental anguish suffered by these concerned individuals was a direct result of feelings of helplessness in the area of bringing comfort and relief from pain and disease to their hospitalized loved ones.

Mary C. was one such person tormented by her feelings of helplessness in relieving the pain suffered by her young son, Bobby. Bobby was 15 and had suffered extensive second and third degree burns in an automobile accident. In the first few weeks of his hospitalization the young man's pain was relieved through the use of narcotics, but a point was reached when the continuation of the drugs that allowed Bobby to be pain-free would have meant his addiction to narcotics, and so the pain-relieving drugs had to be discontinued. Bobby's burns were a long way from being healed and the pain they caused him filled his room with cries and screams begging someone to help him. Mrs. C., who had been at her son's bedside from the first day of his hospitalization, must have suffered mental pain as severe as the physical pain endured by her son when he looked at her through tear-filled eyes and cried, "Mother, help me. Please Mother, do something about this pain!"

Mrs. C. had heard of the course I was teaching dealing with the power and use of the mind in metaphysical healing, and she called to ask for my help. While Bobby's father took up the vigil at his bedside, his mother sat in a classroom with me for two hours. During that time I outlined for her the step-by-step technique that would bring the miracle of metaphysical healing to her son. Bobby's parents had engaged the best medical doctors to care for their son and now they wished to add to this expert medical attention the power and use of their own minds in bringing the miracle of metaphysical healing to Bobby.

Mrs. C. took the several sheets of paper on which I had outlined the miracle technique she and her husband were to use for Bobby's recovery and returned immediately to Bobby's bedside. Not more than five minutes after her return to Bobby's room, both parents began to use the miracle of metaphysical healing for their son. One hour later Bobby dozed off into peaceful sleep for the first time in four days. He slept soundly for four hours and then opened his eyes and spoke with his parents briefly before falling back into a gentle sleep that lasted until the next morning. Bobby's comment during that brief moment of wakefulness brought tears to his parents' eyes, but this time they were tears of happiness.

"Mother, Dad, thanks for helping me. It doesn't hurt anymore. I'm just awfully sleepy."

Mr. and Mrs. C. continued to use the technique for the miracle of metaphysical healing and Bobby continued his rapid progress toward recovery free from pain. The last time I heard from the C. family it was Mr. C. who had told me that Bobby's burns were healing much more quickly than the medical doctors had expected. Prior to the introduction of metaphysical healing, it had been stated by the attending physicians that skin grafts for Bobby would be extensive and would involve several surgical operations. Mr. C. seemed delighted to tell me that the prognosis for his son had been revised and that now, "Bobby will only need one or two minor operations for skin grafts. He hasn't experienced pain since the day we started using the miracle of metaphysical healing. I only wish we had started using those techniques four days earlier. It could have saved Bobby an awful lot of pain."

Mr. and Mrs. C. are not unlike millions of parents who have at one time or another been placed in a situation of believing that they were helpless to aid a sick or injured child. They will never know the pain of that helplessness again. Bobby's parents are well-aware of the fact that the miracle of metaphysical healing is a many-sided gift. It not only brings comfort and relief from pain and illness to the sick, but also brings relief of the pain of helplessness to those who love the patient.

You can use these same miracle techniques that will allow you to bring comfort and health to your loved ones and to free yourself from feelings of helplessness. The miracle of metaphysical healing tapped by the power of energized mind is available to you today in a failproof step-by-step method which you will learn in this very chapter. Your ability to bring metaphysical healing will grow increasingly stronger each time you use this miracle of energized mind.

DISTANCE IS NO OBJECT TO THE MIRACLE OF METAPHYSICAL HEALING

You may find, as many others have found, that it is not always possible to be in the physical presence of a loved one when he or she is ill. You need not let this fact worry you one bit. The power of energized mind and the miracle of metaphysical healing will work just as well for you whether your loved one is in another room or another country. Through the force of energized mind your thoughts carry the miracle of metaphysical healing anywhere in the world. You need not concern yourself about a delay in time any more than you need to be concerned about great distances which separate you and your loved one. Your thoughts that carry the miracle of metaphysical healing will travel with the speed of light since they are powered by the strongest force in the universe—the power of energized mind which emanates from the high self.

Once you have learned the techniques presented to you in this chapter, you will be like a lighthouse which throws its rays of light many miles into the night in order to lead those in peril to safety. You, however, will have a power no lighthouse has ever had, for you will be able to send the light of metaphysical healing completely around the world, if necessary. Reinforced with these techniques, you are by far the most valuable friend any individual could have since you possess the knowledge to bring the miracle of metaphysical healing to that person no matter where he or she might travel.

THE MIRACLE OF METAPHYSICAL HEALING REACHES MORE THAN ONE THOUSAND MILES

Linda J. had been a student in two of my classes where techniques for the miracle of metaphysical healing are taught. Linda was sincere in her desire to master the techniques for metaphysical healing and quickly got into touch with the healing force within herself. She brought the miracle of metaphysical healing to many friends, and many friends of friends. Linda had given many people irrefutable evidence as to the power of energized mind in bringing metaphysical healing to the minds and bodies of others. Linda had one strong opponent to her belief in and practice of metaphysical healing, her sister who lived more than one thousand miles away. She had spent many hours of a one-week vacation at Linda's home criticizing her for her belief in "such a silly thing."

When my phone rang at 11:30 one evening, I was quite surprised to hear Linda's voice on the line. The sound of her voice made it clear that something was wrong, and as she told me why she had called, I understood the reason for her emotional upset.

"My brother-in-law just called me. My sister, Judy, has had a terrible accident. She tripped in the garden and a piece of metal wire pierced her left eye. Bob said the doctors feel she has a 95 percent chance of losing her eyesight in that eye, and won't know until 10:00 in the morning whether or not they will need to operate.''

"I know you're upset, Linda. What can I do to help?''

"You can help me send metaphysical healing to Judy. From what Bob said it will take a miracle to save her eyesight in that eye. He's nowhere near as skeptical as Judy and he asked for my help. He also asked me to call you and ask that you send metaphysical healing also.''

"I'll be glad to help, Linda. I'll start immediately, and you do the same. Please let me know in the morning what the doctors decide.''

We hung up and I began to send the miracle of metaphysical healing immediately. I was sure that Linda was doing the same, and felt that Judy was lucky to have two people using the power of energized mind to bring healing to her injured eye.

Linda and I had agreed to send the miracle of metaphysical healing four times between the time of our conversation and 10:00 A.M. the following morning.

It was 1:30 in the afternoon when Linda rang my phone again. She sounded excited and relieved as she told me of her conversation with her brother-in-law.

"Bob said the doctors cannot understand it, but Judy will not need surgery. It appeared to them that much of the damage had restructured itself overnight and they now feel that corrective glasses will do the job. The doctors arranged for the prescription for the glasses to be filled on an emergency basis and Judy will have them by this afternoon. She's supposed to wear them every day and return to the doctor in one week.''

"That's great, Linda. I'm glad she will not need the surgery. Is there anything else I can do to help?''

"You know there is. Continue to send metaphysical healing and I will, too. The way I figure it, Judy won't even need the eyeglasses for very long.

"I'll call you as soon as I hear from Judy and Bob. Just keep sending that metaphysical healing, okay?''

"Okay, Linda, will do. Let me know as soon as you hear from your sister or brother-in-law.''

Linda kept her promise to call me and one week later at 5:00 in the evening my phone rang and her excited voice bubbled from the receiver.

"You're not going to believe this. What am I saying? Of course, you'll believe it. Judy's eye is 100 percent okay. The doctors are amazed, Bob is amazed, and best of all, Judy is amazed. Wait until I tell you what happened."

"Well, calm down and tell me what happened."

"Bob and Judy had a long talk and decided that they wouldn't even get the prescription for eyeglasses filled. The doctors didn't give them much of a chance for helping her eye, anyway, so Bob convinced her that since metaphysical healing had helped her so far, she should go with it all the way.

"Anyway, when Judy returned to the doctors, they gave her the good news that the glasses had worked. Her eye is 100 percent okay and her vision is just as good as it ever was. When she told them she never had the prescription filled the doctor almost fell over in shock. After blessing her out for not following his orders, he told her he was really glad that her eye was okay, and that however it happened he was glad for her sake."

"That was a little risky of them not following the doctors' orders, Linda. You know I have always said that the miracle of metaphysical healing is to work alongside of medicine, not in place of it. I hope you explain that to Bob and Judy—anyway, I'm awfully glad, too, that Judy's eye is fine."

"Sure I explained about the use of metaphysical healing alongside of medicine. Listen, the two of them are so excited, I think I'll have to explain it again later. I just wanted to thank you for teaching me about the miracle of metaphysical healing and for sending the power of energized mind along with me. Judy is planning to call you herself tomorrow. She wants to learn all she can about metaphysical healing. I know you weren't trying for one, but you have two new students—Bob and Judy."

My two new students, Bob and Judy, have been doing fine for almost a year. They studied the techniques of metaphysical healing and have used the power of energized mind many, many times in their daily life. Judy summed up her feelings in one succinct comment, "It's hard to look with a closed mind through an eye that has had its sight saved through the miracle of metaphysical healing!"

The successful use of the miracle of metaphysical healing in Judy's case gives you clear evidence not only of the fact that distance is no object to the power of energized mind, but also shows clearly that the miracle of metaphysical healing is a potent force in avoiding dangerous and painful surgery. Any physican will tell you that whenever possible it is best to return the patient to health without resorting to surgical procedures. The danger inherent in any surgery is itself great, but just as great is the danger which accompanies the administration of anesthesias.

You can use the miracle of metaphysical healing in order to make dangerous and painful surgery unnecessary for your loved ones. No one likes to face the prospect of undergoing a surgical operation, and through the power of energized mind you have the ability to make such operations unnecessary for those you love.

BREAST SURGERY IS AVOIDED

When Martin L. came to see me he was upset for several reasons. Martin and his wife, Jean, had just learned that she would have to undergo breast surgery for the removal of a non-malignant tumor in approximately two weeks. The presence of the tumor was enough to upset Martin and Jean, but added to that was Jean's fear of the surgery itself and Martin's concern about that fear.

Jean was a housewife and mother and much of her time was devoted to the care of her three children, ages two, four, and six. Surgery for Jean would mean hospitalization for one week followed by a recuperative period of from two to three weeks. Martin's job made it necessary for him to spend two or three nights out of town each week and his wife's hospitalization and recuperation would mean that their three children would need someone to look after them around the clock. Both Martin's and Jean's parents were deceased and they had no relatives living within the state, and they were faced with the fact that they had no likely candidate to look after the children in Jean's absence. All these concerns taken together were making life at this particular time very uncomfortable for both Martin and Jean.

"Well, that's the story, and now I want to know if you will help me. I want you to teach me the techniques for metaphysical healing. I know such healing is possible, but I also know that a person would have to know what they were doing in order to have that healing be effective. I'm willing to do everything necessary to learn how to heal my wife so that she will not have to have breast surgery."

"I have the step-by-step technique written out, Martin, and I only ask that you follow it three times a day.

"When is Jean scheduled to go back to the doctor?"

"She's supposed to go back in three days for her final examination before she enters the hospital."

"I'd like to call me after her visit to the doctors in three days. Between now and the time for that final examination be sure to use this technique three times a day."

Martin left and I didn't hear from him again until the day of Jean's final examination. He called to tell me the good news—Jean's tumor had dissolved and she would not need the surgery.

"I only wish I had known about this technique two years ago when I had to have a hernia operated on."

Martin and Jean have continued to use the step-by-step techniques for the miracle of metaphysical healing with their entire family. They have already begun teaching those techniques to their oldest child and plan that their two youngest children will learn the techniques as soon as they are old enough to understand and practice them.

You can use the same technique to keep your family and loved ones healthy and out of operating rooms. You are never powerless to help a loved one.

YOUR SECRET FOR BRINGING THE MIRACLE OF METAPHYSICAL HEALING TO YOUR LOVED ONES

You will find the step-by-step technique easy to follow and 100 percent effective in its results. Read the technique through twice and then follow the step-by-step failproof instructions.

1. Form in your mind a clear idea of the injury or disease you wish cured through metaphysical healing.

2. Choose a location in which you are not likely to be disturbed and either lie down or sit comfortably in a chair whose back is high enough to support your head.

3. Close your eyes and take a deep breath through your nose following the passage of that breath through your entire body with your mind's eye. Relax your stomach muscles completely

and exhale the breath through your nose. Repeat this breathing technique three times.

4. In your mind's eye form your own motion picture of your loved one's recovery. For example, if your loved one is afflicted with a benign tumor you will allow that non-malignant tumor to take shape in your mind's eye and then through the power of energized mind you will watch as that benign tumor begins to shrink and continues to shrink until it is no longer in existence.

If your loved one has been injured in an accident as was the case with Linda J.'s sister, allow yourself to form in your mind's eye a clear picture of the injury. Now, through the power of energized mind allow motion to be added to your mental pictures and watch as thousands of new cells rush to repair the damaged areas of the body.

5. You are now ready to add sound to your mental motion picture. With the picture of your loved one firmly in your mind's eye, hear that loved one tell you that, "I am completely cured. I am absolutely healthy and without any sickness or injury."

6. Allow yourself to feel the gladness and relief that comes with this loved one's recovery. Accept this recovery as already accomplished for your high self is already bringing your mental motion pictures into actualization.

7. Do not allow yourself to dwell on any negative thoughts or any doubt concerning the effectiveness of this procedure for the miracle of metaphysical healing.

8. Relax for a few moments, allowing yourself to appreciate your own uniqueness and the fact that the power of energized mind works through you to bring the miracle of metaphysical healing to your loved ones.

9. Spend only as much time on this procedure as you are able to give with your full undivided attention. Spend no more time than 15 minutes during one metaphysical healing session.

10. Open your eyes and go about your daily life.

Do not let the seeming simplicity of this technique fool you. The steps outlined allow you to tap within yourself the most powerful force in the universe. You are a born healer and are now in the possession of a step-by-step method which will allow you to bring the gift of metaphysical healing to each and every one of your loved ones.

YOU CAN PREVENT YOUR LOVED ONES FROM BECOMING ILL

You can use the miracle of metaphysical healing to prevent illness as well as to cure it. Once your family has attained perfect health, you can make sure that they maintain that precious gift. Presented with a choice it would seem that preventing illness and injury rather than curing it has been one of the aims of medical science since its conception. The miracle of metaphysical healing allows you, the reader, to make the dream of preventive medicine a reality in the lives of those you love. Everyone who has learned to use the power of energized mind has found that metaphysical healing not only brings the miracle of health to those suffering from illness or injury, but that the miracle of metaphysical healing has kept their family and loved ones in a state of perfect health where even simple maladies such as the common cold no longer afflict them.

Begin now to use the failproof miracle method which allows you to surround your loved ones with a protection no disease or injury can penetrate. Spending only about five minutes of your time each day, the failproof method which follows is your key to keeping your family in perfect health.

HOW TO USE PREVENTIVE MEDICINE THROUGH THE MIRACLE OF METAPHYSICAL HEALING

1. Select a location in which you are not likely to be disturbed. Lie down or sit in a chair whose back is high enough to support your head.

2. Close your eyes and perform the breath exercises as outlined in previous metaphysical healing techniques.

3. Use the mental eye of your mind to create a motion picture of your family and all your loved ones. Include as many people as you like. You cannot overuse your ability to use the miracle of metaphysical healing.

4. In your mental motion picture see your family and all your loved ones in perfect health and enjoying the gifts of peace of mind and happiness. You are to use your mental ear to hear such things as, "I've never felt better in my life," and, "Why it's been years since I've been ill in any way at all."

5. You must not allow yourself to dwell on any negative thoughts concerning the effectiveness of this technique for preventive medicine. Accept the reality of the miracle of metaphysical healing and your high self using the power of energized mind through the miracle of metaphysical healing will keep your family completely healthy, filled with vitality, and overflowing with happiness.

6. Open your eyes and go about your daily life.

You will find that this failproof technique will take about five minutes of your time each day and yet the benefits derived from its use will bring uncountable blessings to all your loved ones. Through these miracle methods you will be able to surround your family and friends with love and health every minute of their lives. Don't waste another minute of your life—begin immediately to use the miracle of metaphysical healing to bring health to all those you love.

three

Metaphysical Healing
Brings Uncommon Cures
for Everyday Sickness and Pain

Did you know that your body is created in such a way that it naturally wants to be healthy? That's right, your body does everything it can through its own power to keep you healthy and pain-free. In a sense pain is not always a bad thing. It is often the intelligence of your body sending out signals that something has gone wrong and your health is in danger. Sometimes your body uses fever to signal you that healing is needed in one or more systems in order that your health may be restored and maintained. When infection strikes at the body, special blood cells rush to the infection sight in order to destroy the illness-producing organisms and aid the body in its natural quest for health. Your body is truly a magnificent creation and only a supreme intelligence could have brought such a creation into existence. That same supreme intelligence also brought your mind into existence, and you may be sure that you are expected to use that mind to aid your body in its natural quest for health.

If you consider the fact that your mind has the power to affect your body and actually restore and replace damaged cells, you can recognize immediately that the mind is even a more magnificent creation than the body itself. Through the miracle of metaphysical healing you have the power this very moment to restore and retain health throughout your body. Remember, your body wants to be healthy and is extremely anxious to take the energy you direct to it through the power of energized mind in order to make that condition of health a reality.

You are now familiar with the great power of energized mind, but your mind also possesses another form of energy known as ultra-mind which is especially effective in bringing uncommon cures for many of the illnesses that affect large numbers of our population. The energy which emanates from ultra-mind is particularly effective in dealing with such maladies as ulcers, arthritis, bursitis, and any other illness which is associated with a great deal of physical pain. The miracle of ultra-mind quiets and rids the body of pain while it restores or replaces body cells.

If you have any doubt as to the great numbers of people who suffer from ulcers, arthritis, or bursitis, you need only give your attention to the communications media for one day. You will be bombarded with ads for patent medicines that promise to alleviate the terrible pains of arthritis, special ointments that are said to alleviate the torment associated with bursitis, and some supposedly wondrous medications that will deal with both at the same time. In seven out of ten movies which deal with life in general, and particularly the life of business people, you are sure to find one or two of the characters who suffer from ulcers. Unfortunately, thousands of viewers who see these movies are also suffering from ulcers and the disabling pain which accompanies them. Cartoons in magazines often poke fun at the man or woman who suffers from stomach ulcers, but the man or woman who finds that he or she is the victim of such an ulcer will find the accompanying pain no laughing matter. With the power of ultra-mind you can bring the miracle of metaphysical healing to yourself and your loved ones not only to rid the body of the pain associated with ulcers, but to heal the ulcer itself.

MAN CURES HIMSELF OF ULCERS AFTER SEVEN YEARS OF SUFFERING

Seven years of suffering with a stomach ulcer had left Richard K. a depleted man physically, emotionally, and financially. Mr. K. had held a top managerial position for 14 years with a major U.S. company. He had developed an ulcer after seven years of stress and constant worry about "getting ahead" in the company. At first Mr. K. thought it would be easy to live with a stomach ulcer and that it would be a small price to pay for the prestige and financial rewards that would be his if he were successful in his company. He was quite successful, and promotion followed promotion at an accelerated rate;

unfortunately for Mr. K. his ulcer was getting worse at the same accelerated rate and the pain he at one time felt would be easy to endure was becoming unbearable.

Richard K. had visited physician after physician who was considered an expert in dealing with ulcers, but despite the expert medical attention, Mr. K.'s ulcer was getting worse instead of better. It became necessary for him to miss a day or two of work each week due to the severe pain and discomfort which he suffered. The lost time made Mr. K. anxious concerning his position and this added stress only served to make his pain worse.

In addition to the severe physical pain and emotional worry concerning his position, Mr. K. had spent a small fortune running from one doctor to another seeking the medication that would stop his pain even if it didn't cure his ulcer.

One of my ex-students who was a friend of Richard's recommended that he speak with me concerning the miracle of metaphysical healing. Mr. K. made an appointment with me with just such a purpose in mind. He made it clear when the day of his appointment finally arrived that speaking with me concerning metaphysical healing was a last resort.

He listened intently while I explained the power of ultra-mind in curing not only pain caused by ulcers, but ulcers themselves. I explained the ultra-mind technique to him step-by-step and he agreed to follow it three times a day. When we parted company, Mr. K. said only that he would let me know one way or the other how the technique worked in his case.

One week later I received a long distance phone call from Mr. K. who was at a large airport on the East Coast. He wanted me to know the technique worked so well that he had been pain-free from the second day he began using it. Now he was on his way to Europe on company business, a trip which only two weeks earlier he did not feel he would be able to make. He was to return in one week and had already made an appointment with a physician for a complete physical and X-rays.

"You'll hear from me again as soon as I complete that physical examination. I just wanted you to know how much better I do feel and how glad I am that I can make this trip myself."

Just as he had promised, Mr. K. telephoned me again ten days later. This time his news was even better.

"The X-rays show that my ulcer is completely healed. I've been taken off my special diet and also I no longer have to take any medication.

"Thank you for sharing the technique of ultra-mind with me. I only wish I had discovered it seven years ago."

I still hear from Mr. K. about twice a year and during our last conversation he informed me that he had received another promotion.

"The promotion has meant more responsibility and more stress, but no ulcers. I've been using the energized mind technique for preventive metaphysical healing every day and I've never felt better in my whole life. I don't know an executive in the world who could not benefit from the use of these techniques.

Executive or not, we are all more alike than we are different. Stress and ulcers play no favorites concerning professions. The same ultra-mind technique that worked so completely for Mr. K. will also work just as completely for you. You can use the technique for yourself or for a loved one with complete confidence that it will bring the miracle of metaphysical healing to the intended recipient of its benefits. Don't make the mistake of suffering unnecessarily or standing by while someone you love suffers the pain of ulcers. Learn the following miracle technique and you will find living in a world filled with stress and tension a great deal easier.

YOUR ULTRA-MIND TECHNIQUE
FOR THE CURE OF ULCERS

Read the technique through at least twice and then follow the step-by-step instructions which will guarantee you and your loved ones freedom from ulcers.

1. Select a location in which you are not likely to be disturbed. Lie down or sit in a chair whose back is high enough to support your head.

2. Close your eyes and for a moment let yourself be aware of your own intake and outflow of breath. Make no attempt to control your breathing process, only watch it with undivided attention for one minute. You will find that this concentration will help you to relax completely.

3. Take a deep breath through your nose and with your mind's eye follow that breath as it flows throughout your entire body

and finally comes to rest in the area of your ulcer. Repeat this breath technique three times.

4. Form a picture in your mind of the ulcer from which you or your loved one suffers.

5. Repeat the following words mentally to your high self: "I recognize myself to be a magnificent human being. I acknowledge the fact that my mind is all-powerful in bringing into actualization that which I want to come about. I will that all my energies be directed to and conducted through my ultra-mind power. I will that the power of ultra-mind act with all its force to restore or replace all ulcerated cells in my body and deliver to me through the miracle of metaphysical healing the gift of perfect health."

6. Create a motion picture across the screen of your mind and see yourself or your loved one with the physician who has been treating the ulcer. Through the miracle of ultra-mind add sound to your mental motion picture and hear the physician state, "The X-rays show that your ulcer is completely healed. You can stop the special diet and medication and eat anything you like."

7. Again watch your breathing for one minute without any attempt to control it. Repeat the following words to yourself mentally: "Every second of this day the power of my ultra-mind will send the miracle of metaphysical healing to all ulcerated cells in my body. Though my conscious mind may be engaged in other matters, my ultra-mind will concern itself continuously with my return to perfect health."

8. Open your eyes and go about your daily life.

You will find that this miracle technique practiced three times daily will completely heal any ulcer no matter how severe it may be. The miracle of metaphysical healing directed through ultra-mind cannot fail to restore ulcerated cells and place your body in a condition of perfect health.

If you or someone close to you suffers the pain of bursitis then you know that the torment brought about by this affliction is no laughing matter. The pain of this inflammatory disease has been the cause of many sleepless nights for thousands upon thousands of individuals. Those individuals have suffered needless pain and lost sleep unnecessarily. If you are one of the people who make up the large numbers of those suffering from bursitis or if one of those individuals is a relative or a friend of yours, realize that at this moment you have the power not only to rid yourself and your friends and relatives of the pain of bursitis, but to cure the inflammatory condition itself. Decide now that you will not suffer another moment, but will begin immediately using the power of ultra-mind to replace bursitis and all its accompanying pain with your birthright—perfect health.

You have more power available to you in the area of your high self than is stored in all the atomic and hydrogen bombs that have ever been created upon this earth. Add to this the fact that your power channeled through the areas of ultra-mind and energized mind for the purpose of metaphysical healing is a creative force and you will see once again that not to use this miracle power of metaphysical healing would be a senseless and almost criminal act. Remember, the more you use the miracle of metaphysical healing the stronger your powers will become. You cannot run short of the power of ultra-mind nor of the power of energized mind. Your continuous use of these faculties of your high self will cause them to become more accessible to you, and their miracle power will continue to grow without limitations.

With such miracle power made available to you through the techniques of metaphysical healing you are obliged to keep yourself and loved ones in a condition of perfect health. In this book is all the knowledge you will ever need to conquer any disease or injury and it is vital that you exercise the miraculous power of your high self through using the miracle techniques for metaphysical healing daily in your life.

WOMAN WHO SUFFERED FOR TEN YEARS WITH BURSITIS CURES HERSELF THROUGH THE POWER OF ULTRA-MIND

When I first met Katherine T. she was 50 years old. She had suffered from bursitis in both shoulders for ten agonizing years. Katherine told me that she had been aware since her early twenties that every individual has the power to restore health to the sick and injured. What Katherine lacked was the knowledge of the miracle techniques which would allow her to tap the limitless source of power within herself.

"Unfortunately, knowing that I have this power to heal myself isn't enough. I don't know how to go about it."

Katherine was 100 percent correct, for to know that a home is completely equipped with electric lights and yet not know how to find the switch that turns them on will leave a person completely in the dark. Katherine was determined to find the switch that would allow her to tap the miraculous powers of ultra-mind and bring the gift of metaphysical healing to her pain-racked body.

Since Katherine T. already recognized the fact that she was by nature a healer, I was able to begin immediately teaching her the step-by-step method through which the miracle of metaphysical healing would restore her to perfect health. She listened intently as I went through the step-by-step instructions that Katherine was to use three times a day. She was one of the most determined individuals I have ever met and during the hour we talked she did not utter one negative statement. Because of her lack of negativism the road to perfect health would be much shorter for this charming woman who had suffered physical torment only because she lacked a knowledge of the miracle techniques that would allow her to tap the limitless powers which she knew her high self possessed.

After providing Katherine with a step-by-step method for curing bursitis, I asked only that she keep me posted as to her progress. It did not surprise me in the least to receive word from Katherine only three days after our meeting that the pain she had suffered for ten years had left her after the second time she performed the miracle method for the cure of bursitis and had not returned since. It was also no surprise when she stated, "I was real lucky in getting an appointment with my doctor right away. He examined me, took some X-rays, and told me that all evidence of bursitis had left me. I don't know who was happier, him or me!"

The last time I heard from Katherine T. she had offered her services as a volunteer worker at a hospital in her hometown. She explained, "I really intend to let other people in on this miracle of metaphysical healing. There must be thousands just like me who know they have the power to heal themselves, but just don't know how to go about it. Working as a volunteer in a hospital, I should be presented with many opportunities to share these techniques with patients who express an interest."

If you or a loved one has suffered the painful inflammation of bursitis simply because you did not know how to bring the miracle of metaphysical healing to yourself, it is time your suffering stopped. The miracle method that worked for Katherine T. in curing her bursitis will work just as well for you and your loved ones. The same step-by-step method which Katherine used is given in this chapter so that you, too, may benefit through tapping the power of your ultra-mind and bringing a state of perfect health to your body through the miracle of metaphysical healing.

Don't delay another minute! You possess a natural ability to bring health to your body and combined with the miracle method given in this chapter you need never suffer the pain and inflammation of bursitis again, nor spend another sleepless night due to the agony of this condition.

YOUR MIRACLE METHOD FOR CURING BURSITIS

Read the instructions through carefully at least twice and then follow the step-by-step instructions that will bring the miracle of metaphysical healing into your life.

1. Select a location where you are not likely to be disturbed. Lie down or sit in a chair whose back is high enough to support your head.

2. Close your eyes and for a moment watch your breathing without attempting to control it.

3. Take a deep breath and immediately relax your stomach muscles. Let your mind's eye follow the breath through your body and bring the breath to rest in the area where the bursitis inflammation exists. Repeat this exercise three times.

4. Repeat the following words to yourself mentally: "I will the miracle power of my ultra-mind to concentrate all the energies of metaphysical healing in the areas of my body afflicted with bursitis. Through the power of ultra-mind I will that all cells of my body damaged by bursitis are now completely restored to perfect health."

5. In your mind's eye create your own motion picture complete with sound. Let this mental motion picture enact a visit to your doctor's office. See yourself seated before your physician (if you are sending the miracle of metaphysical healing to a loved one, then picture the loved one seated before his or her physician) and repeat the following conversation mentally to yourself: "I'm happy to tell you that from your physical examination and the X-rays we have taken I have found that your bursitis condition is completely healed. I don't quite understand how

this has happened, but I am very pleased for you that it has happened.''

''Thank you very much, doctor. It feels wonderful to be free of the pain and discomfort of bursitis, and I am very thankful for the gift of health.

6. Take a deep breath, extending the diaphragm and immediately relax your stomach muscles. Allow your consciousness to follow this breath through your body, bringing it to rest once again in the area of your body afflicted by bursitis. Repeat this breathing exercise three times.

7. Once again, watch your breathing with no attempt to control it. Relax completely and repeat the following words to yourself mentally: ''Through the miracle of metaphysical healing directed by the miraculous force of my ultra-mind, my body is restored to a completely healthy condition. All inflammation and cellular damage due to the affliction of bursitis has been replaced with completely healthy cells.''

8. Open your eyes and go about your daily life.

You will feel the miraculous powers of this step-by-step method for curing bursitis immediately. In a very short period of time you will find yourself free not only of the pain caused by bursitis, but also free of the inflammation and affliction of bursitis itself.

You will also find that the practice of this miracle technique will bring new relaxation and new health to all the muscles in your body. Your ultra-mind is a source of limitless power that is at your continual disposal day or night. Whether you use this miracle power to bring healing and health to yourself, or use it to bring healing and health to a loved one, you will find that it will never fail you. When you call on the miraculous powers of ultra-mind in order to bring health to a diseased body, there is no such thing as failure. Success is the only possible outcome in any situation where the power of ultra-mind is introduced by you.

ARTHRITIS SURRENDERS QUICKLY TO THE POWER OF ULTRA-MIND

Thousands of people of all ages are at this moment caught in the crippling effects of arthritis. In addition to a restriction in movement, these people also undergo severe pain for which medical doctors can do very little without running the risk of having the patient addicted to a habit-forming pain reliever. The power of ultra-mind does not restrict itself to the alleviation of pain, but always goes to the origin of the pain itself in order to bring new health to diseased areas of the body while at the same time leaving the suffering individual pain-free. What sensible individual would be content with freedom from pain alone, when that individual has the power within himself to bring about a complete cure from the disease or injury causing that pain?

If you or one of your loved ones happens to be one of the thousands suffering the pain and restriction of arthritis, decide now that you will be free not only from the pain, but also from the arthritic condition itself. Ultra-mind is the road by which you can bring the gift of health and freedom of movement to yourself and your loved ones. You must not delay another minute, for you possess at this very moment all the miraculous power necessary to rid yourself and your loved ones of all traces of arthritis. To continue one more day without using the miracle of ultra-mind which has been placed at your disposal would be to take this wonderful gift which is yours by your very nature, and fling it back into the face of the giver of all gifts. You have not only the right, but the obligation to use this miraculous force of ultra-mind to bring healing to yourself and to your loved ones. I'm sure you have heard it said many times that "God helps those who help themselves." You have been given everything necessary to help yourself to reach a condition of perfect health and it is your obligation to use what has been given to you in order to bring healing and health to any organ or limb afflicted by disease or injury.

WOMAN CURED OF ARTHRITIS IS ABLE TO LEAVE HER WHEELCHAIR

The fact that arthritis is no respecter of the young was brought home to me with striking force when a young mother first visited me two years ago. Susan R. was 32 and had been confined to a wheelchair for two years due to the effects of crippling arthritis. The arthritic condition from which Susan suffered affected not only her legs, but also involved her spine to a great extent. As the mother of two young children, ages six and four years, Susan had discovered that keeping up with a young family while riding in a wheelchair is not an easy matter.

"My four year old son, Greg, is full of life and thinks there is nothing better than running as a means of travel. Even if my chair had a motor, I couldn't possibly keep up with him."

Lack of mobility was not the only cross brought to bear on Susan and her family through the effects of arthritis. "Sometimes I could kick myself for being cross with my family. My husband can understand, of course, that at times the pain is so bad that I bite anyone's head off just for smiling at me. It's not that easy to get the two boys to understand that at times I'm in such pain I'd growl at the angel Gabriel himself if he appeared before me."

Susan wanted to be free from the pain and restriction she suffered from arthritis, but she also wanted her family freed of the restrictions placed upon them because she was unable to be the wife and mother that she felt her family deserved. She had been told by many physicians that there was no hope for her condition, and that the best she could hope for was to adjust to her limitations and expect her family to do the same. As time passed and the pain got worse and one restriction was piled upon another for Susan, she decided that she would be healed in spite of the fact that medicine could offer no cure to her or even the promise of a possible cure in the near future. Susan was determined that she would be free from arthritis, and free from her wheelchair.

This determined frame of mind was evident the entire hour of our first meeting. "I just know something can be done about this arthritis. I've heard you on different radio shows, and I believe in what you say about the fact that the mind can cure the body. What I want you to do now is teach me how I can use my mind to get rid of this arthritis."

We discussed the metaphysical healing technique that would restore Susan's body to perfect health, and Susan agreed to follow all instructions for the use of her ultra-mind in order to cure herself of arthritis. When Susan left she smiled broadly and said, "The next time you see me I'll be walking."

Susan proved to be a woman of her word. Three weeks after our first meeting I was at the university catching up on some paper work when I was interrupted by a knock on the door. The door opened and in walked Susan R. smiling broadly. "Well, you were right and so was I. The miracle of metaphysical healing sure is powerful stuff. When are you going to let more people in on this miraculous power?"

We talked for a while and Susan explained to me how she had

returned to her doctor as soon as she found that she could stand and walk. "You could have knocked him over with a feather. I bet it took him at least two days to get his mouth closed. He was in such shock I thought I'd have to call a doctor for him."

Susan did most of the talking telling me of her plans for the future and how wonderful it was to be able to walk again. We both laughed as Susan told me of Greg's surprise when he found that he could no longer outrun his mother.

As Susan was leaving she paused at the door for a moment, smiled like the proverbial cat, and asked, "Do you know anyone who wants to buy a used wheelchair?"

When I last heard from Susan she was a den mother and chasing not only Greg, but a whole troop of young boys and was happy to report that she could outrun anyone in her troop. She still had her wheelchair but it had not been used in two years except by her two sons who enjoyed turning it into an imaginary race car. She told me to forget about finding a buyer for the chair, "With the miracle of metaphysical healing available to people, why would anyone want to buy a wheelchair?" Susan had a good point.

The identical technique that allowed Susan R. to use the power of her ultra-mind to bring the miracle of metaphysical healing to her own life is available to you in this chapter. Follow the step-by-step instructions daily and you, like Susan R., will be cured from arthritis. You can add yourself to the growing numbers of ex-arthritis victims starting today.

YOUR BLUEPRINT FOR THE CURE OF ARTHRITIS

Follow the instructions listed below and repeat this miracle technique three times a day.

1. Select a location in which you are not likely to be interrupted. Lie down or sit in a chair whose back is high enough to support your head.

2. Close your eyes and watch your breath for a moment without attempting to control it.

3. Take a deep breath from the diaphragm and immediately relax your stomach muscles. Allow your consciousness to follow the circulation of the breath throughout your body, bringing it to rest in all areas of your body afflicted with arthritis. Repeat this breathing technique three times.

4. Repeat the following words to yourself mentally: "Through the power of ultra-mind I will that every arthritic cell in my body be healed immediately. I will that the miracle of metaphysical healing restore or replace each of my cells that has been touched by arthritis.

"I release all resentments that I may have felt towards others in my life, and I will that these people be directed in their life to their own highest good."

5. Create a mental motion picture and allow it to flow across your mind's eye. See each part of your body that has been afflicted with arthritis return from a swollen condition to normal size. Add the miracle of motion to your mental movie and see any limbs that have been previously restricted in movement due to arthritis, moving freely. Allow this mental motion picture to run across your mind's eye for from one to two minutes.

6. Now add the miracle of sound to your mental movie. See yourself in your doctor's office and hear your physician say to you, "My examination and the X-rays that I took indicate that you no longer have any traces of arthritis. I cannot explain how it happened, but you are completely cured from your arthritic condition."

See yourself leaving the doctor's office, but pausing to say, "Thank you, doctor. You don't know how glad I am to be rid of arthritis. I'm looking forward to doing all the things I couldn't do before due to the pain and lack of motion in my limbs because of arthritis."

7. Take a deep breath from your diaphragm and relax your stomach muscles immediately. Allow your consciousness to follow that breath, permitting it to come to rest in all areas of your body afflicted by arthritis. Repeat the following words to yourself mentally: "Through the power of ultra-mind each breath I take during the day brings new energy which restores and replaces all cells in my body afflicted with arthritis. Enriched with the miracle of metaphysical healing each breath I take speeds me on my way to complete and perfect health."

8. Watch your breath for one minute without any attempt to control it. Allow yourself to be aware of the relaxation that has come to rest upon your entire body.

9. Open your eyes and continue your daily life.

You will notice that step four of this miracle technique of ultra-mind for the cure of arthritis instructs you to release all resentments that you may be holding against any person. This is an extremely important step in your cure from arthritis. Each time you hold a resentment toward another human being you rob yourself of energy that would normally go to the upkeep and maintenance of your physical and emotional health. No grudge is more important than your own perfect health, and anyone would be a fool to allow a grudge to stand in the way of a cure from arthritis.

Medical science has been aware of the effects of resentment in the formation of arthritic conditions for many years. A Boston physician, Dr. Loring T. Swaim, who was an instructor for 20 years at Harvard Medical School, specialized in orthopedics and arthritis, and spoke frequently as to the effects of resentment and grudges in causing and aggravating arthritic conditions. Dr. Swaim and many other physicians have been convinced for many years that a patient, in order to be free of arthritis, must also be free of resentments.

In another chapter of this book you will learn how to rid yourself of negative thinking and all forms of resentment. Remember, no grudge or resentment is more important than your cure from arthritis!

THE SLIMMING EFFECTS OF ULTRA-MIND

A prevalent condition in the lives of many people today, and one that has been found by medical doctors and scientists to be an aggravating factor if not the outright cause in many diseases afflicting the body and the mind, is that of obesity. The person who allows himself to amass extra pounds of body weight has placed himself where high blood pressure and heart disease have a better than average chance of gaining a foothold on his body. Medical science has stated many times that obesity actually shortens the expected life span of any individual. This is to say nothing of the fact that the daily life led by the severely overweight individual often finds them significantly lacking in energy and the butt end of many jokes aimed at "fat people" in our society.

We are all familiar with the fact that many varieties of diet foods and beverages are on the market and are advertised as aids in helping an individual lose weight. We are all just as well-aware of the fact that many comedy situations have been created for TV and movies concerning the overweight individual who finds it "impossible" to lose the extra poundage he has accumulated. In almost any bookstore we can easily find anywhere from ten to 20 books that deal with "easy" methods for losing weight. It's a sad statement, but true, that thousands of overweight individuals have purchased one diet book after another in an attempt to find the special diet that will work for them, and yet still find themselves to be many pounds overweight.

You need never find yourself in such a position. For you, it will not be necessary to search through hundreds of books on special diets in order to find a technique that might work for you. In this very chapter you will learn the miracle technique of ultra-mind that cannot fail to work for you and will not only melt pounds off your body, but will keep them off. The miraculous power of ultra-mind which you will follow in an easy step by step method is also at your disposal for aiding your loved ones in losing unhealthy poundage that does damage to their physical and emotional health.

Whether you desire to lose ten pounds or 100 pounds, the miraculous power of ultra-mind is the reducing method you have been looking for. Your ultra-mind contains everything needed to melt ugly fat from your body. Now the technique that will allow you to tap this miraculous power of ultra-mind is at your fingertips.

WOMAN LOSES 90 POUNDS THROUGH THE USE OF ULTRA-MIND

When I first met Margaret D. one and a half years ago, no one could possibly have guessed that she was only 27 years old. Margaret was five feet, three inches tall and weighed an overwhelming 200 pounds. She had tried diet after diet with little or no success. She had joined expensive health clubs hoping that their exercise methods would enable her to lose the extra weight that was endangering her physical health, dampening her emotional outlook, and playing havoc with her social life. The health clubs, like the diets Margaret had tried, had little or no effect on the numbers staring her in the eye whenever Margaret stepped on a scale. Even the expert directions of two physicians whom Margaret visited in hopes of losing weight were not successful in shrinking her extra poundage by more than three pounds in four months.

Margaret was about to give up when a friend suggested that she speak with me concerning the role of the mind in losing unwanted pounds. To paraphrase Margaret, she had tried everything and nothing had worked, and she didn't really have much hope that any technique I could teach her would work where so many other techniques had already failed.

"You have no idea how frustrating it is to try so hard and still look like a blimp. All those stories about fat, jolly people are a bunch of baloney. Do you have any idea how hard it is just to find clothes that will fit?

"I've even tried going to a hypnotist in order to lose weight. That didn't work either."

It didn't take a psychiatrist to realize that Margaret's outlook concerning weight loss was deeply pessimistic. The first thing that was needed was to get Margaret to believe in her own abilities shedding the cloak of pessimism she had woven out of so many disappointments. We talked for 45 minutes before Margaret was in a frame of mind where discussing the exact instructions she was to follow would do her any good.

Margaret listened intently and her ears really perked up when I told her that it would not be necessary for her to exclude any particular food because it was high in calories or carbohydrates. "You see, Margaret, the power of ultra-mind will regulate your appetite for you. You just won't want as much to eat, and the foods you do particularly crave will be foods relatively low in calories and carbohydrates. The miracle of metaphysical healing will not only cure your obesity, but will also cure your over-zealous appetite."

It was agreed that Margaret would visit me again in one month. In the month before her return visit she was to follow the instructions given to her for the use of ultra-mind in bringing the miracle of metaphysical healing to an obese body and an appetite that desired enough food to feed at least three individuals. Margaret showed up for our next meeting carrying a bathroom scale under her arm. It was evident that she had lost a good amount of weight, but it was also evident that she still had some way to go. As she placed the scale on the floor and stepped on it she said, "Take a look for yourself. Do you see that? One hundred and seventy pounds. I've lost 30 pounds in one month! Thirty pounds and I'm not even going hungry!"

We talked for a while and Margaret wanted to know if following the exercise four times a day instead of three times would not be better. I assured her that the instructions she had been given needed no improvement and she agreed to follow the exercises three times a day. We would meet again at the end of another month and even though Margaret didn't mention it, I knew that she would have the bathroom scale with her at our next meeting.

The month seemed to fly by and again Margaret was keeping a pre-arranged appointment carrying her bathroom scale. She had chosen to wear the dress she had worn for our appointment the previous month, and it was quite obvious that the dress was many sizes too large for her. Again Margaret put the scale on the floor and stepped on it asking me to come and see what numbers would call out her weight. She now weighed 130 pounds!

I could not help but smile to myself when Margaret spoke with me in a voice heavy with concern. "I'm getting to the point now where I may be in danger of losing too much weight. Let's see; I lost 30 pounds the first month and 40 pounds this month, if I lose either of those amounts again I'll be too skinny!"

Mixed with the concern in Margaret's voice was also a large amount of joy over the fact that she had to be concerned with being too skinny! I explained to Margaret that the high self could be directed through the use of the miraculous power of ultra-mind to stop weight loss when a desired weight had been reached. Margaret decided that she wished to weigh 110 pounds. This meant that she needed to lose only 20 more pounds in order to attain her goal.

After I had given Margaret instructions on how to direct the higher self to stop the weight loss process when the desired weight goal had been attained, she left stating that she was in a hurry since her social life had picked up greatly since her body weight had gone down.

Margaret did not make another appointment, but was to come to visit me when her body weight had reached 110 pounds. She paid that visit three weeks later carrying the same bathroom scale she had brought with her on her second visit. As she stepped on the scale the numbers 110 announced the fact that Margaret had reached her desired goal concerning her body weight. In less than three months' time Margaret had lost a total of 90 pounds. She had been reshaped from a woman weighing 200 pounds and looking twice her age into an attractive young woman of 27 who weighed 110 pounds. Her social life had also reshaped itself and Margaret had begun dating a handsome young attorney on a regular basis. She looked wonderful and according to Margaret, "I've never felt better!"

Six months ago Margaret married her handsome young attorney and moved with him to another state where he had been offered a partnership in a thriving law practice. Her body weight has remained constant at 110 pounds, while her optimistic outlook on life and the degree of happiness she experiences has continued to increase. For Margaret D. the loss of 90 pounds opened the door to an entirely new life.

You now have the opportunity to lose as much or as little weight as you would like. The miracle technique which Margaret used to lose 90 pounds is presented for you here, and also presented for your use is the instruction on directing the higher mind to stop the weight loss when your desired weight has been attained. Whether you use this technique to bring the miracle of metaphysical healing to yourself or to a loved one, you will find it a failproof method for the loss of weight. Begin now to use the power of your ultra-mind in the following miraculous method and never worry about being over-weight again.

YOUR ULTRA-MIND TECHNIQUE FOR WEIGHT LOSS

Perform this exercise three times a day. If you are more than 40 pounds over your desired weight, do not concern yourself with the directive to the higher mind at this time. If, in order to reach your desired weight, you need lose 40 pounds or less, then incorporate the directive to the higher mind as the fourth step in your miracle technique for weight loss.

1. Select a location where you are not likely to be disturbed. Lie down or sit in a chair whose back is high enough to support your head.

2. Close your eyes and for one minute watch your breath without any attempt to control it. Be aware of the relaxation flowing through your entire body.

3. Take a deep breath extending your diaphragm and relax your stomach muscles immediately. Allow your consciousness to follow this breath through your entire body, watching as it is absorbed in part by all your body cells. Repeat this breath exercise three times.

4. Repeat the following words to yourself mentally: "Through the miraculous power of my ultra-mind, I direct that my physical body will begin this very moment to lose weight. I direct that with a loss of weight my body will attain and maintain a

condition of perfect health. I further will that the intelligence of my high self will direct that this weight loss shall be proportional in that I shall lose weight only in areas where weight loss is needed.''

5. Repeat the breath exercises as outlined in number three, but now allow your consciousness to follow the distribution of breath to the areas of your body where weight loss is most needed.

6. Repeat the following words to yourself mentally: ''Through the miraculous power of ultra-mind I will that the miracle of metaphysical healing shall also be brought to my appetite, and that I shall desire the most nutritious foods for my body and only in amounts that my body can use for the attainment and maintenance of perfect health.''

7. For one minute watch your breath again with no attempt to control it. Allow yourself to be aware of the great feeling of relaxation that flows through your entire body.

8. Open your eyes and go about your normal daily life.

SPECIAL DIRECTIVE TO THE HIGH SELF

4-A. Repeat the following words to yourself mentally: ''Through the miraculous power of ultra-mind I direct my high self to continue my physical weight loss until I have reached a weight of (here insert your desired body weight) pounds. When I have reached this desired body weight, my high self will direct that weight loss be discontinued and that my chosen body weight will be maintained and that.all systems of my body shall be in complete and perfect healtn.''

This special directive to the high self is to be used only when a person's excess body weight does not exceed 40 pounds. It is to be inserted in the fourth step of the instructions given above so that the instructions above numbered ''4'' will become number ''4-B'' and will be preceded by the special directive to the high self.

You will be surprised at the speed and ease at which your body loses physical weight while it gains a new vitality and reaches a level of optimum health. With the use of the miracle technique given above you and your loved ones need never be concerned about overweight again.

SINUS PROBLEMS BECOME A THING OF THE PAST

If you or one of your loved ones has ever suffered the pain and discomfort of a sinus headache accompanied by swollen eyes and difficult breathing, you are well aware that sinus problems are no laughing matter. It makes no difference whether your sinus problem is caused by hay fever or an infection or other allergies, the pain which accompanies that problem is often so severe as to incapacitate its victim. If you have sought medical help for your sinus problem, chances are that you have been told that there is no such thing as a cure for chronic or acute sinusitis. The medical person who gave you this bit of information was speaking the truth, that is, he was speaking the truth if he was concerned only with a cure as brought about through conventional medical treatment. As wonderful as medical science is today, and despite all the advances it has made, it can offer no medical cure to the sinus sufferer. True, certain prescription drugs may be prescribed that will in some small way decrease sinus congestion, but the drugs themselves can often have unpleasant side effects and cannot offer a cure from sinus problems.

If you have suffered one sinus headache in your life, you have suffered enough from this painful inflammation that affects millions of people throughout our world. Now through the miraculous power of ultra-mind you need never suffer another sinus headache or other accompanying sinus problems. The miracle power of ultra-mind can reach far beyond the frontiers already touched by medical science and bring metaphysical healing to you or your loved ones who suffer from sinusitis.

WOMAN CURES HERSELF FROM SINUS PROBLEMS

Ruth N. had suffered from chronic sinus problems and sinus infections since she was five years old. As a mature woman of 35 she could remember the many trips to different physicians from the time she was a child and continuing on for 30 years. Her parents had taken her to physicians specializing in the treatment of ear, eye, nose, and throat, to allergists, and to physicians who specialized in diagnosing the patient's problem. Once in a while Ruth was able to obtain some relief from a new medication prescribed by a particular physician but soon her body would develop a tolerance for the particular drug and it would no longer be effective in alleviating the pain caused by her sinus problems.

In addition to a long list of medications which had been administered to Ruth since her childhood, her parents had spent a fortune on doctors' fees and prescriptions by the time she was 19 years old.

"I think my parents would have been glad to spend the money if only I had been able to gain some real relief from the treatments and medications. Any relief I got was only temporary and the money my parents had to put out was fantastic when you add it all up."

I met Ruth through a mutual friend, and at first she was hesitant to ask my help in regard to metaphysical healing for her sinus problems. She finally explained her circumstances to me and asked if I would teach her to use the miracle of metaphysical healing in order to cure herself from chronic sinus infections and rid herself of the terrible pain associated with them. I agreed to teach her the technique of ultra-mind designed for the cure of sinus problems and she agreed to follow the instructions explicitly.

Two weeks later I received a phone call from Ruth N. telling me that she had been back to her doctor and that the X-rays had shown her sinuses to be completely clear of infection and congestion. She had not had a sinus headache, post-nasal drip, or swollen eyes since she had begun using the ultra-mind technique for the cure of her sinus problems.

"My doctor is an eye, ear, nose and throat specialist, and I wish you could have seen his face when he saw my X-rays. He's taken me off all medications and I've never felt better in my whole life.

"Thanks a lot for teaching me about the miracle of metaphysical healing. I have three friends whom I met in my doctor's waiting room who suffer from the same type sinus problems I used to have; they want to learn the ultra-mind technique, too. They'll be calling you in a day or two. Thanks again for your help."

On the following day I did receive three phone calls from the three women Ruth spoke of concerning their sinus problems. I shared the same ultra-mind technique with them and in two weeks all three were dismissed by their physician with a clean bill of health. I hear from the four every so often and they have formed what they jokingly call the Ex-Sinus Sufferers Sorority at whose meetings "no sniffling is allowed."

Sinus congestion and sinus infection can be a terrible irritation and bring almost unbearable pain to those who suffer its results. You need never be in such a situation, for you now have available to you the same technique that worked for Ruth N. and her three friends. Follow the instructions given in this chapter for the cure of sinus problems and sinus infections and you will find that your sinus problems are a thing of the past.

YOUR ULTRA-MIND TECHNIQUE FOR THE CURE OF SINUS PROBLEMS

Repeat the following technique three times a day. You will find it a failure-proof method for the cure of sinus infection and all sinus problems. Don't suffer a minute longer from sinus irritation; begin now to use the power of your ultra-mind to bring the miracle of metaphysical healing to yourself and your loved ones.

1. Select a location where you are not likely to be disturbed. Lie down or sit in a chair whose back is high enough to support your head.

2. Close your eyes and for one minute watch your breath with no attempt to control it. Allow yourself to be aware of the complete relaxation which flows through your entire body.

3. Take a deep breath extending the diaphragm and allow your consciousness to follow that breath through your entire body bringing it to rest in the sinus cavities of your head.

4. Repeat the following words to yourself mentally: "Through the miracle power of ultra-mind all the energies of my high self are directed to bring about a condition of perfect health throughout the sinuses of my body. With the force of ultra-mind I direct that all cells of my body affected in any way by sinus problems or sinus irritations be at this moment completely restored or replaced and that all my sinuses will be in a condition of perfect health and in perfect harmony with all other systems of my body."

5. Create a mental motion picture and allow it to run across your mind's eye. See yourself (the sinus victim) with your physician and hear him speak the following words, "My examination and the X-rays have shown that your sinus problem is completely cleared up. There's no evidence of sinus irritation and so we will discontinue medication."

See yourself leaving your doctor's office and pausing at the door long enough to say, "Thank you very much, doctor. You don't know how glad I am to be rid of sinus problems for good."

6. Take a deep breath extending the diaphragm and immediately relaxing the stomach muscles. Follow the breath with your consciousness and allow it to come to rest in all the sinuses of your body. Be aware of the fact that all cells affected by sinus irritation are utilizing the energy and healing power of ultra-mind and are at this very moment restoring themselves to perfect health.

7. For one minute watch your breath with no attempt to control it. Allow yourself to be aware of the total relaxation which flows through your entire body.

8. Open your eyes and go about your daily life.

This ultra-mind technique for the cure of sinus problems cannot fail you. Perform this exercise three times a day by following the step-by-step instructions, and you will never be bothered with sinus problems again.

In this chapter you have been made aware of the miracle techniques which will allow you to tap your ultra-mind and bring the miracle of metaphysical healing to the many maladies which plague mankind. You as an individual who is aware of the existence of your ultra-mind and the techniques by which you can direct its miraculous power need never suffer from pain, disease, or injury again. You are now able to bring the miracle of uncommon cures to everyday sickness, injury, and pain.

four

You Can Bring the Miracle
of Metaphysical Healing
to the Mind and Emotions

You have already learned how the mind can play an important part in bringing sickness to the body. You have also learned that the miracle powers of ultra-mind and energized mind can restore damaged cells and bring health to any body illness or injury.

There are cases, of course, where an individual's mind or emotions may become ill and make it impossible for that person to lead a happy and healthy life. There are many patent drugs on the market that promise to ease the tension of everyday stress and strain. There are hundreds of other drugs known as tranquilizers which physicians prescribe for patients suffering from emotional illness or upsets which do not seem to respond to patent medications. Whether you have suffered such emotional upsets yourself, or are aware of a loved one who has been the victim of emotional illness, this chapter will be of great interest and benefit to you. It offers you all the necessary techniques for tapping the miracle power of energized mind and ultra-mind for the purpose of bringing calmness and health to anyone who suffers from emotional illness or upset.

You may feel that emotional illness and pain is very different from physical illness and pain, but actually they have much in common. You and every other human being on this earth can be faced with only one problem. That problem may present itself in many different ways; emotional illness, physical suffering, and depression and unhappiness are only several of the ways that problem becomes manifest in the life of mankind. The basic problem of mankind is that countless individuals do not recognize the infinite power available to them within their own mind. If you and your loved ones are not aware of the fact that all things are possible to you through the miracle power of energized mind and ultra-mind, then you fall prey to the major malady of mankind—the malady of not realizing the miraculous power which dwells within you by virtue of the fact that you are a member of the human race.

You, as a reader of this book, already know that the miracle power of metaphysical healing is available to you 24 hours a day. You know that there is no physical disease, illness, or injury that you cannot heal with the miraculous force of your own mind. You also know that there is no emotional illness, mental disease, or emotional upset that can withstand the miraculous force of metaphysical healing. In this chapter you will learn how to tap the miracle force of ultra-mind and energized mind in order to bring calmness and freedom from all stress and tension into your life.

If you have been one of the many individuals who has daily or at times taken tranquilizing drugs or patent drugs which promise to bring calmness to those who suffer from nervous tension, know now that you never need to take another medication in order to bring tranquility into your life. The miraculous power of metaphysical healing is so strong that no psychological crutches will be needed at any time in order to be and feel healthy. Psychological crutches are for mental cripples, and you and every man, woman, and child on this earth have received as your birthright a power of mind so miraculous that nothing which stands in the way of your mental, emotional, or mental health can withstand its force. The miracle techniques which follow in the pages of this chapter will help you make that birthright an infinitely important part of your everyday life.

MENTAL AND EMOTIONAL ILLNESSES HAVE MANY FACES

Emotional illness can show itself in your life and in the lives of your loved ones in many ways. Individuals who have allowed their lives to be touched by alcoholism, nervous stuttering, nervous twitches and tics, and just plain "jittery nerves" are all victims of emotional upset or mental illness. Indeed, mental and emotional illness can be so severe at times as to actually paralyze its victims. If your life or the life of one of your loved ones has been touched by any disease condition which has its roots in the emotional make-up, know that at this very moment you have the power to bring peace and tranquility back into that tortured life. If you have ever stood by and watched, feeling helpless as a friend or relative had their life torn down around them through alcoholism, know that at this very moment you have the power to cure not only yourself from alcoholism but also to bring that cure through the miracle of metaphysical healing to all relatives and friends.

THROUGH THE MIRACLE OF METAPHYSICAL HEALING A MAN IS CURED FROM HIS DESIRE FOR ALCOHOL

The family of Walter J. had suffered much over a ten-year period due to his excessive alcoholism. Walter had succeeded through the excessive use of alcohol not only in bringing terrible misery and suffering to his own life, but had succeeded in making the lives of his wife and four children a miserable reflection of his own life.

Walter J. had been a successful advertising executive for 20 years, and during that time he had provided his family with a beautiful home and many luxuries. Walter and his wife had planned that each of their children would be able to attend college if they so desired and had set up savings accounts in order to insure that the money would be available when each child was ready to enter higher education. He had been the perfect husband and father for 20 years, drinking only moderately and then only at social gatherings. Like that of so many others in our society, Walter's drinking problem began when he received a promotion that meant not only recognition for his past work but brought with it increased stress and tension from his future work. Unable to cope satisfactorily with the new tension in his life, Walter began drinking not only at social gatherings, but at all hours of the day and night.

At first Walter was still able to keep his drinking under control, or so it seemed. As the days wore on the new tension that had been introduced into Walter's life began to wear on him more steadily and he began to drink more heavily. In two years time he had changed from a man who drank only one or two drinks at parties to a man who was drinking every day and ending every night with his mind in a drunken condition. His wife and children pleaded with him to cut down on his drinking, for it was obvious that it was affecting not only his emotional health but his physical health as well. Their pleading seemed to have no effect for Walter's drinking became even heavier and more frequent. It surprised no one but Walter when at the end of his third year in his new position he was suspended from his job and told to seek medical help for his drinking problem.

Walter seemed sincerely shocked as he related the facts of his suspension to his wife. He was certain that alcohol held no power over him and that his suspension must be the result of in-company jealousy. Walter continued to drink just as heavily as he had before he was suspended from his job, and refused to see a physician as was suggested by his company. The additional unstructured time available to him was spent downing drink after drink in an insane attempt to show that alcohol was not an addiction for him.

Suddenly Walter J. seemed to change. He had always been a pleasant and considerate man, but now as his alcoholic intake increased his disposition seemed to change for the worse. He became argumentative and seemed to delight in needling his own family concerning areas that were particularly sensitive spots for them. After two months of such treatment Walter's family was at a position where some decision had to be made for the sake of their own mental and physical well-being. Mrs. J. talked with Walter and tried to explain the detrimental effects his drinking was having on his wife and children, not to mention the effects it had already had on his own life. Walter only insisted that he only drank on occasion and then only to ease the tension which he as head of the household had to bear. In the following month Walter's children and wife continued to plead with him to stop drinking by seeking professional help. He vetoed the idea of joining Alcoholics Anonymous, outwardly laughed at the idea of consulting a physician, and ended by forbidding that the subject of his alcoholic rehabilitation ever be mentioned in his home again.

Finally when his family could endure no more pain his wife and children left him. Instead of being rocked to his senses by the loss of his family, Walter continued his devotion to the bottle and his fast trip physically and mentally downhill. His family were gone, his mortgage was overdue, his bills were stacked up unpaid, his company had told him they would not hold his position indefinitely, he had lost much weight, he spent his waking hours in emotional pain and still he seemed unable to take the steps that would put him back on a sober path to a happy life.

It was Mrs. J. who came to see me and discuss her husband's situation. She and her children were willing to do anything they could to help Walter regain the large portion of himself which he had lost to alcohol. Mrs. J. was a firm believer in the miracle of metaphysical healing and had seen it work many times in cases of physical illness or injury. Now the cure she was interested in obtaining for her husband was not only for a physical malady, but one from an emotional and psychological addiction to alcohol. Walter's wife and children agreed to follow a step-by-step technique which I presented to them so that they might bring the miracle of metaphysical healing to their father. They followed the technique faithfully and at the end of seven weeks Walter phoned his wife in order to tell her that he had decided to give up drinking entirely. Alcohol no longer made him feel good, but instead seemed to increase all his tension, stress, and was even leading to physical discomforts.

"I can't explain it, but I just don't have the desire for alcohol that I had before. I know now that I was addicted to it and I can't fully understand why all of a sudden I don't have the same drive towards it that I had only months ago."

When Walter had gone two additional months without a drink and had been back at his job for two weeks, he and his family were reunited. The J. family was much luckier than the majority of families torn by alcoholism. Through the miracle of metaphysical healing the J. family had brought the gift of healing to Walter J. and to itself. The family has not been bothered by alcoholism since and they give full credit for the miraculous cure of Walter J. to the miracle power of metaphysical healing.

YOUR STEP-BY-STEP MIRACLE METHOD FOR THE CURE OF ALCOHOLISM

It is unfortunate but true that in 99 out of 100 cases of alcoholism a cure through the use of metaphysical healing will be brought to the victim through the efforts of family and friends. The unfortunate part is not that the victim of alcoholism is aided by family and friends, but that the victim is seldom able to do much in the way of helping himself. In recognition of this fact the technique provided here for the miracle cure of alcoholism through the use of metaphysical healing is directed primarily to be used by those who would help a friend or a relative receive healing from this destructive addiction. It would be extremely beneficial if organizations dedicated to the rehabilitation of alcoholics would use this technique at every meeting in order to bring help and rehabilitation to the thousands of alcoholics in our country alone.

This technique may also be used by the reformed alcoholic who wishes to remain a non-alcoholic and decides to use the force of metaphysical healing to keep himself free of tension and stress that might lead back down the road to alcoholism.

The technique that follows may be used by individual members of a family or may be used by a family as a group. The combined use of individual and family participation for the purpose of bringing metaphysical healing is strongly encouraged.

The following steps are guaranteed to bring the miracle of metaphysical healing to your friends and loved ones. Follow the steps faithfully every day and watch the miracle of metaphysical healing transform the twisted lives of friends and relatives so that they might share a fulfilling existence utilizing their talents and gifts to the utmost.

1. As with all techniques for the miracle of metaphysical heal ing it is important that you find a location where you are not likely to be disturbed. Lie down or sit in a chair whose back is high enough to support your head.

2. Close your eyes and allow your consciousness to be aware of your breathing. Do not attempt to control your breathing but only watch it in your mind's eye. As you become aware of the intake and outflow of breath, be aware of the relaxation that flows through your body as your mind watches the process.

3. Take a deep breath through your nostrils, extending the diaphragm as you inhale, and in your mind's eye watch that breath as it travels throughout your body and finally ends its journey in the area of your brain. Repeat this breathing process three times and with each inhalation be more aware of the increased relaxation flowing through your body.

4. Repeat the following words to yourself mentally: "I have filled myself with the miracle energy of metaphysical healing and now will direct that energy for the purpose of bringing to my friend (or relative) a complete and lasting cure from an addiction to alcohol."

5. Begin to produce your mental motion picture which will aid in bringing the miracle of metaphysical healing to your friend or relative. For a brief second recognize your friend or relative in

the situation in which he or she is addicted to alcohol. Now begin to send the energy of energized mind by seeing your friend or relative politely turning down an invitation to have a drink. In your mind actually hear the words of the invitation and the polite refusal by your friend or relative.

See your friend or relative walking by liquor stores, looking in the window smiling to himself, and walking by without stopping for a purchase.

See your friend's family and close friends gathered around him and create a conversation in your mind similar to the one given below.

"It's wonderful not to need alcohol any longer. I don't understand it, but I have no desire any longer to drink. I feel so much better, too, no longer tense or on edge."

"That's wonderful. You don't know how great it is to see you happy again."

Allow your mental motion picture to see your friend or relative completely cured of a desire for and addiction to alcohol. Allow yourself to hear the conversation between your friend or relative and other members of the family or other friends.

6. As in step three, take a deep breath through your nostrils, extending the diaphragm, and completely relax your stomach muscles. In your mind's eye watch the breath as it moves throughout your body and focuses finally in the area of your brain. Allow yourself to be aware of the relaxation that flows through and around your body and mind.

7. Repeat the following words to yourself mentally: "Through the miracle of metaphysical healing infinite amounts of healing energy are being focused on (here give the name of the person to whom you are directing the miracle of metaphysical healing) and are bringing this individual to freedom from tension, stress, and a freedom from an addiction to and desire for alcohol."

8. Open your eyes and go about your daily life.

Repeat this exercise three times a day. This is your failproof technique for bringing a cure from an addiction and desire for alcohol to your friends and loved ones.

We are all aware that an addiction to alcohol is a serious problem in this country, but there are also other emotional and mental upsets which bring conditions into the life of an individual and the life of a family which are unpleasant and unhealthy. The miracle of metaphysical healing is also designed to bring a freedom from all mental and emotional upsets through bringing the gift of metaphysical healing to the mind and emotions of all mankind.

Few, if any, would argue against the fact that the pace which mankind has set for itself on our planet and especially in our country is one that surrounds man with stress, tension, and places him in the position of being the victim of his own emotional and mental conflicts and confusions. The national media presents us with stories of individuals who have suffered serious physical, occupational, and social damage as a result of emotional and mental stress.

The humor of comedians often deals with an individual who because of nervous tension has developed a "nervous twitch" and has become the proverbial ineffectual "nervous wreck." Prescription tranquilizers and patent medications designed to bring temporary relief to the individual suffering from tension are not cures for the stress that plagues mankind. The miracle of metaphysical healing brings the only cure possible to any individual who has become a victim of mental and emotional stress and conflict. Every individual has the power within himself to bring this gift of metaphysical healing to his own life and also to the life of a friend or loved one. This chapter makes available to you the techniques that are failproof in freeing you and all friends and relatives from the stress, confusion, and tension that can wreak havoc in an individual and family life.

WOMAN CURES HERSELF OF NERVOUS STUTTERING

When I had just entered my teens we lived next door to a family whose only son, a 16 year old boy, suffered from serious nervous stuttering. I can remember feeling embarrassed for this young man when for one reason or another he appeared at our home to borrow a cup of sugar or convey an invitation from his parents and was faced with the difficult task of making the purpose of his visit vocal. It was very difficult not to give him the words he sought for so intently as his emotional pain became more obvious, as did his reddening face and scuffling feet. It is unfortunate that at the age of 13 I had not formulated strong convictions or techniques regarding the miracle of metaphysical healing and the ways it could have been used in such a situation. It pains me somewhat to state that I do not know at this time of the whereabouts of this young man who was my neighbor for two and one half years. Perhaps he will read this book or someone will tell him about the miracle of metaphysical healing so that he can receive a cure now that I was unable to offer him so many years ago.

There are thousands of people in this country alone who suffer from nervous stuttering or other forms of speech malfunction due to emotional or mental stress. The miracle of metaphysical healing offers these thousands of individuals a cure from the physical manifestations they endure and the mental tension and emotional stress that underlies their apparent problem. One such individual sought my help two years ago.

When Karen R. first introduced herself to me, it was an introduction replete with difficulties for Karen. Karen was a petite, attractive young woman of 23 who suffered from a serious stuttering problem. Her speech would progress perfectly for four or five words and then pauses would begin to occur with greater and greater frequency. During these pauses it was apparent to anyone present simply from watching Karen's face that she was making a painful attempt to frame her thoughts in vocal speech.

I honestly could not tell you how long our first visit lasted, since I lost track of time holding to my resolve that I would not put words into Karen's mouth. Eventually Karen got her story out and asked for help through the miracle of metaphysical healing. Karen's personal history was in many ways similar to the histories of many individuals who suffer from nervous stuttering. She was the oldest of three children and, from what she had been told by her family, she had begun to stutter at the age of four and one half. At that time the family did not feel the stuttering was severe enough to warrant medical attention or corrective speech classes. Mr. and Mrs. R. had always felt that Karen was a sensitive child and was unduly nervous and would outgrow this nervousness with the coming years. Unfortunately, the coming years saw a worsening of Karen's stuttering problems and her family decided to seek the help of a speech therapist.

From the time Karen was seven until she reached her fifteenth birthday she attended speech classes regularly and practiced home exercises vigorously for the purpose of ridding herself of her stuttering problem. To quote Karen, "Nothing seemed to help. Instead of my stuttering getting any better, it seemed to get worse. I began to dread school since even when I knew the answers having to express them verbally was even more painful than having the class think I was just dumb." This dislike for the painful circumstances presented by a classroom situation reflected itself in Karen's refusal of an offer from her parents to send her to college. Karen was determined that she would not put herself in another classroom situation and decided to find a job that would allow her "to keep her mouth shut."

She found a job with a national company as a sewing machine operator. Karen had kept that same job for five years and was employed with that company when she came to see me. She had received increases in salary, but never increases in responsibility. Despite the fact that Karen knew the operations of her department inside out, it was obvious that she would never be promoted to a position supervisor, since that position meant a needed ability for verbal communication. Verbal communication or not, Karen had had it! She was bored with doing the same thing day in and day out and had also begun to realize that the waste of her fine mind would only make her more unhappy. She was willing to do anything necessary in order to be cured from her stuttering and she wanted to start right away.

Karen's eagerness was a great help to me in helping her to understand the scientific facts behind the miracle of metaphysical healing. She took the sheets of paper I had given her outlining the step-by-step method by which the miracle of metaphysical healing would be introduced into her life for the purpose of curing her stuttering and the underlying nervous tension that caused it and promised to carry out the exercise faithfully three times a day. She was to keep me posted of her progress and she was to use the telephone in order to do this.

One week after our first meeting Karen telephoned me and it was easy to recognize from listening to her that her stuttering problem had already greatly improved. Her words flowed much more easily and the pauses were not quite so frequent as they had been at our first meeting. She would continue the exercises and keep me up to date.

The next telephone call I received from Karen came two weeks after her first call. If I had not known of her previous stuttering problem, I never would have guessed that she ever suffered such a situation. Her words flowed freely and there were no pauses that were obviously painful times of search for adequate vocal expression.

"How about this! Isn't it wonderful? I haven't stuttered in ten days. This may seem silly to you, but two nights ago I recited the Gettysburg Address for my family and did it without once stuttering.

"Thank you so much for sharing the miracle of metaphysical

healing with me. I can promise you that I will also share it with anyone who needs the help it can provide."

Two months after that phone call Karen was made supervisor of her division of the company for which she worked. Despite this recognition and an increase in salary Karen decided that she would like to attend college. She made application and was accepted at one of the country's top universities for the purpose of pursuing a course in secondary education. She is still attending school and plans to teach as soon as she graduates. "Imagine that, me teaching, when just a little while ago I would never have gotten up in front of two people to speak, let alone an entire classroom full of students."

The miracle of metaphysical healing has changed Karen R.'s life completely and has enabled her to become a more fulfilled human being. This same miracle of metaphysical healing will work for you and your loved ones just as quickly as it worked for Karen R. It remains only for you to learn the step-by-step technique that will allow you to tap the powers of energized mind already flowing within you so that you will be able to bring the miracle of metaphysical healing into your own life and the lives of others. There is no way that you can possibly fail if you follow the step-by-step method given in this chapter. The miracle power of your own energized mind will free you from all nervous, mental, and emotional tension and cure you from all outward manifestation of those tensions. Begin now to use this miracle technique which will provide a cure from any speech malfunction.

YOUR MIRACLE CURE FOR SPEECH MALFUNCTIONS AND OTHER NERVOUS HABITS

Repeat the following exercise three times a day and you will quickly find yourself free of all nervous tension and nervous habits arising from mental and emotional stress.

1. Choose a location where you are not likely to be disturbed. Lie down or sit in a chair whose back is high enough to support your head.

2. Close your eyes and for a moment watch your own breathing. Give your attention to the intake and outflow of your breath with no attempt to control it. Be aware of the relaxation which flows through your body as you watch your breathing process.

3. Take a deep breath through your nostrils and immediately relax your stomach muscles. Allow your consciousness to follow that breath through your body and bring it to rest in the area of your brain. Repeat this breathing exercise three times, allowing yourself to be aware of the increased relaxation which flows through your entire body and mind.

4. Repeat the following words to yourself mentally: "I am a magnificent human being. Through the power of energized mind I now possess the ability to cure myself and my loved ones of all physical and mental or emotional illness and upsets."

5. In your mind's eye begin to form your own mental motion picture. (This exercise may be used with any nervous habit, but for the sake of example we will use here the speech malfunction of stuttering.) See yourself surrounded by your friends and loved ones, speaking with them freely and with no hint of stuttering or painful pauses. See their faces reflect the astonishment of hearing you speak so eloquently when in the past you were a serious stutterer.

In your mind's eye allow the conversation between you and these people to take place. Hear their words expressing astonishment at your freedom from speech malfunction and their great joy that you have received this miracle cure.

6. In your mind's eye create a mental motion picture which will include you and a professional in speech evaluation. See yourself and your doctor or speech pathologist discussing your cure from speech malfunction. Again see astonishment expressed on the face of the medical expert with whom you are consulting and hear the words of that expert state that you have been cured of a speech malfunction and that despite the fact that he cannot explain the cure scientifically, he is happy that you have received its benefits.

Hear yourself thank this person and then move on to the next step in this exercise.

7. Take a deep breath through your nostrils and immediately relax your stomach muscles. Allow your consciousness to follow the path of this breath throughout your body and allow it to come to rest in the area of your brain. Repeat this breathing exercise three times. Allow yourself to be very aware of the relaxation that flows through your mind and body.

8. Open your eyes and go about your daily life.

With this failproof technique there is no need for you or any friend or loved one to suffer from nervous or emotional or mental tension or the physical manifestations of such tensions. You are a born healer and with this technique you have the secret necessary to free yourself and your loved ones from any nervous habit. There is no mental or emotional stress so strong that the miracle of metaphysical healing is not stronger; there is no nervous habit so entrenched that it cannot be cured through the miracle of metaphysical healing. Don't waste another moment of your life or watch another moment of the life of a loved one wasted because of mental or emotional strain and the physical manifestation this strain can take in an individual life. Begin today to live free from all nervous habits and all mental and emotional stress or tension.

EMOTIONAL STRESS CAN HAVE A PARALYZING EFFECT

It has already been pointed out many times in this book that the mind rules the body for good or ill. Through the miracle of metaphysical healing and the powers of energized mind and ultra-mind you can be sure that your mind controls your body for good, restoring it and maintaining it in a state of perfect health. It may or may not surprise you to learn that the mind can have such a detrimental effect on the body as to produce not only sickness and pain, but to actually immobilize the body and paralyze it. Many well-known psychiatrists have worked with a psychological condition known as conversion hysteria. An individual suffering from conversion hysteria is a perfect example of the effects of negative emotions on the body. Feelings of guilt or fear experienced mentally may be denied by the mind and take their effects on the body paralyzing an arm or a leg or even the entire individual. Anton Mesmer and Sigmund Freud worked with individuals suffering from conversion hysteria, and it is unfortunate that neither of these gentlemen was attuned to the miracle of metaphysical healing so that their patients might have been cured safely and quickly not only from symptoms but from underlying causes.

It is seldom today that we see the term "conversion hysteria" applied to any patient. You might encounter such a diagnosis in an old war movie where a soldier so frightened at the prospect of battle finds that he is unable to move either of his legs. The soldier actually becomes paralyzed by fear and negative emotions.

You don't have to view an old war movie to know that negative emotions and emotional upsets are taking their toll even today. Human beings have allowed their bodies to suffer the consequences of negative emotions and emotional upsets since the beginning of time. People have experienced blindness, loss of speech, deafness, and partial and total paralysis as the result of mental stress and fear. It's a sad fact that large numbers of people today are beset by these same circumstances due to the fact that they have not learned how to use the miracle power of their energized mind as a healing force for all mental and emotional stress.

DAVID L. USED HIS ENERGIZED MIND IN ORDER TO CURE HIMSELF OF PARALYSIS

Most of us would agree that a young man of 19 who is physically attractive and extremely personable and intelligent would have a lot to look forward to in his future life. If you had met David L. on his nineteenth birthday I am sure those thoughts would have flowed through your mind in respect to him. David had been a star on his high school basketball team and since his high school graduation he had enrolled in a course for computer mechanics. He finished the course with flying colors and, following a pattern of success, got a job with a large national company with excellent prospects for promotions. It seemed that David's future was assured and with that fact in mind David had become engaged to his high school sweetheart.

Seven months after David had begun his new job he received a letter that changed the course of his life. The letter began with the word "Greetings" and David had been drafted into the Army. It was no secret that people were being killed in Viet Nam every day, but David had always refused to take part in conversations touching on that subject. The very idea of physical combat petrified him and now it looked as if David would soon find himself on the front lines in a war he didn't even like to think about. Now one letter had forced David to think seriously concerning Viet Nam and combat, and each thought petrified him just a little bit more than the previous one.

He passed his Army physical with flying colors and was to report for basic training in two weeks. It had only been ten days since David had first received his draft notice and yet everyone around him had noticed the change in his personality. It was unlike David to be withdrawn and unfriendly and yet he hardly spoke to any of his friends at work or to his family at home. He had not spoken with his fiancé in five days and when she called his home he would instruct his mother to say that he was not in or was unable to come to the telephone. His parents tried to talk to him but he closed them out, too, and it seemed as if David had retreated into a world where no one else was allowed to enter.

Ten days before he was to report for active duty David did not appear at the family breakfast table. Certain that he had overslept, his mother went upstairs to check on him and was shocked to find David lying in his bed staring at the ceiling.

"Mother, I can't move. I don't know what's happened, but I can't move at all."

David was rushed to a hospital and after numerous tests by his family physician and neurological experts brought to his case for consultation, it was determined that there was no physical reason for David's paralysis. No physical reason, and yet David was truly paralyzed. His freedom of movement was limited to opening and closing his eyes and to speaking. David used his freedom to speak to tell his father to be sure the Army knew of his condition so they could cancel his draft notification.

After three weeks in the hospital and consultations with neurosurgeons and psychiatrists, David was sent to his home by ambulance where he would spend the next five and one half years of his life confined to his bed.

When David was almost 25 his mother came to visit me and asked about the miracle of metaphysical healing as a possible cure for her son. It was through the complete history that she gave and through talking with David later that I learned of the facts presented above concerning the circumstances leading to David's paralysis. After we spoke together for about an hour, it was agreed that I would visit David the next day and speak with him concerning metaphysical healing and the miracle power he possessed in his own energized mind. During my visit with David he was quite receptive to the idea that through the miracle of metaphysical healing he would be able not only to move again, but to move about freely just as he had before the onset of his paralysis. It was agreed that he and his mother would both perform the miracle steps that would bring David back to the full use of his body. They were to use the power of energized mind in the miraculous video-medic technique, the same technique outlined for you later in this chapter.

For the next two weeks David and his mother performed the miracle technique three times a day by following the step-by-step method outlined for them. They were to use the miraculous video-medic technique in order to bring their mental motion pictures into actualization.

Two and one half weeks after my visit to David's home, I received a phone call from Mrs. L. asking me if I could come to their home immediately. She assured me that it was of the utmost importance, so I left immediately for the L. home. When I entered the front door, I was pleasantly surprised by David himself who walked over to me and wrapped me in his arms for a big hug. Actions spoke all the words necessary, David's paralysis was completely cured.

When the excitement died down a little, David and I were able to talk over a cup of coffee. "You know, Evelyn, I realize now that part of the reason my paralysis lasted so long was the fact that I couldn't forgive myself for being afraid in the first place. I know that the fear I experienced was the original cause of the paralysis, but my own guilt at being afraid is what kept it lingering for five and a half years.

"If it wasn't for the video-medic technique and the miracle of metaphysical healing, I hate to think of how many years longer I would have been pinned to that bed by my own mental and emotional confusion.

"I know I can't change the past, but you can bet I'm going to do an awful lot about the future. I plan to enjoy every moment of life and to use the miraculous power of my energized mind in order to bring good things to myself and to everyone around me."

What could I say when David had said it all so well? As I was leaving David assured me that he would keep in touch to let me know just what he was doing to make his promise to himself a reality. He was determined to use the miracle of metaphysical healing to bring the blessing of health to all those with whom he came in contact.

You will no doubt agree that it was a shame that David L. spent an unnecessary five and one half years of his life completely paralyzed by emotional conflict leading to fear and guilt. It is important that you also realize that no matter how many years of his life David may have wasted, the number one issue for David now was what he would do with the rest of his life. None of us can make progress toward a better future if we spend our time beating ourselves mentally for our past mistakes. Perhaps one of the most valuable lessons David learned was that of forgiving himself for showing a human failing. That same lesson is important for you and the miraculous video-medic technique which follows will help you to learn that lesson now.

YOUR VIDEO-MEDIC TECHNIQUE FOR THE CURE OF EMOTIONALLY-INDUCED PARALYSIS

Repeat the following miracle steps three times a day in order to bring freedom of movement to yourself or to the body of a loved one.

1. Select a location where you are not likely to be disturbed. Lie down or sit in a chair whose back is high enough to support your head.

2. Close your eyes and watch your breathing for a moment. Allow yourself to be aware of the intake and outflow of breath without making any attempt to control it. Be conscious of the relaxation which flows through your body becoming stronger every moment.

3. Take a deep breath through the nostrils and allow your consciousness to follow the flow of that breath throughout your body, bringing it to rest in the area of your head. Repeat this exercise three times, each time taking a breath through your nostrils, immediately relaxing your stomach muscles, and following the breath through your body, allowing it to come to rest in the area of your head.

4. Repeat the following words to yourself mentally: "Through the miracle of energized mind, the miraculous force of metaphysical healing is flowing through my body this very moment. (If you are using the miracle of metaphysical healing for another person, insert the individual's name in place of the word "my" throughout this exercise.) It is bringing new tranquility to my mind and emotions and creating within my mind and soul a condition of inner peace."

6. Take a deep breath through your nostrils, extending the diaphragm as you inhale and then relax your stomach muscles completely. For a moment focus all your consciousness on the inner feeling of peace which exists within you this very minute. Allow yourself to be fully aware of the calmness which permeates your very being.

7. Repeat the following words to yourself mentally: "From a position of complete tranquility and through the miraculous force of energized mind, I willingly release all feelings of emotional upset, tension, guilt, and resentment and will that these negative emotions be replaced immediately with the miracle of metaphysical healing."

8. Create your own mental motion picture across the screen of your mind's eye. (Remember that if you are using this technique to send metaphysical healing to another individual, insert that person's name wherever appropriate.) See yourself with complete freedom of movement and with no evidence of previous paralysis.

Use the miracle of your video-medic technique to see yourself surrounded by friends and relatives whose faces show astonishment at your complete recovery from your paralysis. Add to this mental motion picture the quality of sound. Mentally hear yourself engaged in conversation with friends, relatives, and your doctor concerning your complete recovery from paralysis. Hear your friends and relatives saying, "I'm so happy for you. It's wonderful to see you up and around again. One would never know that you had ever been paralyzed."

Now use your video-medic technique to place yourself in the presence of your physician. Hear your physician say, "I'm very happy for you. In spite of the fact that we knew it was nothing physical that was causing your paralysis, there didn't seem to be anything conventional medicine could do to restore you to free movement. You seem so much calmer now and so much happier, it's no wonder the paralysis has left you."

"Thank you, doctor. I appreciate your sharing in my excitement about my recovery."

9. Repeat the following words to yourself mentally: "Even when my conscious mind is engaged with other matters, my high self through the power of energized mind will be continuously flooding my being with the miracle of metaphysical healing in the form of peace and tranquility. Mental stress and emotional tension will remain things of the past for me for my high self will keep me constantly attuned to my highest good."

10. Open your eyes and go about your daily life.

This is the same miracle technique that worked for David L. and it will work just as well for you and your loved ones. Just as your physical body inclines itself toward health, so also do your mind and emotions strive for a state of perfect balance and harmony. With the miracle of metaphysical healing and the force of your energized mind you will be able to live in a constant state of inner peace free from emotional stress and mental conflict. To assure that you and your loved ones will live a constant life of inner peace, perform the following exercise every day. It will bring the blessing of constant mental and emotional health into every facet of your daily life. You have already lived too long without this miraculous technique, so begin now to make inner peace your constant companion.

HOW TO GIVE YOURSELF AND YOUR LOVED ONES THE ULTIMATE GIFT—PEACE OF MIND AND INNER TRANQUILITY

Perform the following exercise once a day. This miracle method is guaranteed to make inner peace and tranquility a habit for you and your loved ones.

1. Select a location where you are not likely to be interrupted. Lie down or sit in a chair whose back is high enough to support your head.

2. Close your eyes and for a moment watch your breath without attempting to control it. Allow your awareness to follow your intake and outflow of breath, and become increasingly attuned to the relaxation which is spreading through your body and mind.

3. Take a deep breath through your nostrils, extending your diaphragm as you inhale. Immediately relax your stomach muscles and allow your consciousness to follow the breath through your body bringing it to rest in the area of your head. Repeat this breathing exercise three times.

4. Repeat the following words to yourself mentally: "Through the miracle of energized mind my high self is constantly aware that the essence of my being exists in perfect harmony and peace at all times. I will that this knowledge be constantly referred to all aspects of my being. I am now and will continue to be at perfect peace within myself. No words or circumstances can

disturb my inner tranquility for it is an essential component of my very nature."

5. Take a deep breath through your nostrils extending your diaphragm as you inhale. Relax your stomach muscles completely and allow your consciousness to follow the breath as it travels through your system and comes to rest finally in the area of your head. Repeat this breath exercise three times. With each new inhalation be more aware of the relaxation which flows through your entire being.

6. Repeat the following words to yourself mentally: "Whether I am by myself or in the presence of one or two other individuals or in the midst of a crowd, I am and will continue to be perfectly at peace within myself. I will that my own inner peace will flow forth from me bringing its gift of tranquility to all with whom I come into contact."

7. Open your eyes and go about your daily life.

Remember that when you are using this technique for a specific friend or loved one, you are to insert that individual's name in all appropriate places. If the friend or loved one for whom this technique is used is suffering emotional or mental pain or is the victim of mental stress or emotional anguish, perform the offered exercise three times a day. There is no way this miracle technique can fail. It will bring inner peace to anyone for whom it is performed.

Once your friend or loved one has received the gift of metaphysical healing for their mental or emotional upset, you need only perform the exercise once a day on the individual's behalf in order to make tranquility a habit for that person.

With the miracle techniques presented to you in this chapter, you need never again suffer from tension or stress. Along with your birthright of perfect physical health you may now claim your second birthright—freedom from all mental and emotional conflict, and infinite inner peace.

five

You Can Add a Touch of Color
to the Miracle
of Metaphysical Healing

Have you ever wished you lived a more colorful life? Which of us would not have our feelings hurt if we heard someone describe our personality as "colorless"? Whether or not you have realized it before, color has always played an important part in your life. Descriptions and phrases using color as essential components in conveying their meanings have always been abundant in our society. Undoubtedly you have worked or attended schools in buildings where special attention is paid to color schemes in order to make efficiency of purpose easier to attain within the building. The "institutional green" used by many companies and schools on the premise that the color green is a calming color is well-known to most of us. Which of you has ever known a person whose bedroom was painted or wallpapered in a brilliant red color?

The science of psychology has long recognized the importance of color in the lives of human beings. Advertising companies use color psychology oftentimes in advertising campaigns and packaging of products so that the prospective buyer's eye will be caught and his attention held in order to make a sale more likely. The next time you are in a large supermarket, take the time to notice how many packages make predominant use of the colors red and yellow in order to catch the customer's eye.

Did you know that color is even important in your diet? Several large food processors and manufacturers have experimented with the use of color as a possible addition of sales appeal to the customer. One world-wide soft drink manufacturer regularly experiments by adding food coloring to a world-wide accepted soft drink. The effect of the added food coloring, despite the fact that it does not alter the taste of the soft drink one bit, is to lead the taster to the conclusion that the soft drink is no longer palatable and the statement that he would not purchase such a soft drink were it to be offered on the market.

If you are the type who likes to conduct your own experiments, I have a suggestion for you based on an actual event in my own life. Like many of you, I am the oldest in my family, and one day my younger sister decided to bake a cake for the family. It just so happens that I love cake, candy, cookies, and all sorts of confectionary goodies, but the cake that Eilene baked was too much for me. Eilene had followed all the instructions on the cake mix box and then decided to add her own creative touch. The creative touch my eight year old sister decided to add was almost an entire bottle of forest green food coloring. She topped it all off by stretching her creativity to the icing and used another bottle of food coloring to turn vanilla icing a brilliant orange. My family did its best to appreciate that cake, but to be very truthful it stayed in the cake plate and still holds the endurance record for any cake in our household. If you keep in mind the fact that I am a confessed cake-o-holic, the strength of this statement becomes even more understandable. The color of the cake turned everyone off!

You are invited to try such an experiment for yourself if you need further proof of the importance of color in the daily life of every human being. With the help of food coloring you can serve such delicacies as royal blue mashed potatoes, bright orange cauliflower, and passionate purple vanilla pudding. Try the experiment or take my word for it; it will go over like the proverbial lead balloon.

Color has a special place in your life as it has in the life of every human being on our planet. Just as important is the fact that every color is unique unto itself in the properties it possesses and the effects it has on human beings. Color can not only turn someone off, it can also turn a person on, and turning you on to good health through the use of color in the miracle of metaphysical healing is the purpose of this chapter. With the information and techniques presented to you here, you will be able to use the miracle of metaphysical healing in order to color yourself the picture of health. To paraphrase an often used cliché, the miracle techniques presented to you here will allow you to "color the roses back into your own cheeks and the cheeks of your loved ones."

The uniqueness of each color became particularly apparent to me during the nine years of my life that I was blind. (My recovery from blindness, epilepsy, and a paralyzed right arm through the use of the miracle of metaphysical healing will be discussed in Chapter six.) Color has something special to offer you on your road to perfect health. Philosophers often talk about archetypes which may be considered universal blueprints for every category of a thing in existence. For example, every chair belongs to a category of chairs, and for the category of chairs there is a universal blueprint or archetype of chairness. Extending this idea to the concept of color, we can state that for everything in our world bearing the color red there is a universal blueprint for redness itself. The archetype, or universal blueprint, redness has its own essential properties which allow it to offer you benefits which no other color can promise. The same may be said for the universal blueprint of blueness, greenness, yellowness, whiteness, and so on all the way down the line until every color is encompassed by its universal blueprint. You might think of this archetype, or universal blueprint, as the special properties which come together to make the color what it is. For instance, without the universal properties which are present in the idea of blueness itself nothing would be colored blue; and without the universal properties which are present in the idea of redness itself nothing would be colored red. It is the universal blueprint of a color which gives the color its strength and special identity. It is your knowledge of these universal blueprints of colors which you will gain in this chapter that will allow you to use these special properties in bringing into your life or the life of a loved one the miracle of metaphysical healing.

THE ROLE OF COLOR IN THE MIRACLE OF METAPHYSICAL HEALING

You will soon be able to use a rainbow of colors which will lead you to a more precious treasure than the proverbial pot of gold. The miracle techniques presented to you in this chapter will allow you to use the special properties of color in order to bring the miracle of metaphysical healing to yourself and your loved ones and keep you constantly in a state of perfect health. Which human being would not agree that the gift of flawless health is worth far more than any treasure of gold and silver? Who is not aware of the tragedies that have touched the families of millionaires who, despite their tremendous monetary fortunes, could not buy healing or health for themselves or their loved ones? No amount of money, or "long green," could buy the miracle of metaphysical healing presented to you in this book.

Since every color is unique, it stands ready to aid you in its own special way. Each color has its own vibratory pattern and ·its own special energy to offer you in bringing the miracle of metaphysical healing to yourself and your loved ones. Colors, like snowflakes, are all different. Some offer you increased energy while others bring you the gift of tranquility, and still others the special energies which fight infection. Through the use of your energized mind you can surround yourself with the energies of the color that offers you the quickest road to perfect health. Aided by your high self you can also select clothing of the colors which will be of greatest benefit to you in the area of metaphysical healing. You need not worry about complicated formulas to memorize or special color charts to follow; the miraculous techniques presented to you in this chapter are beautiful in their simplicity and yet unequaled in the magnificent power they place at your disposal. You cannot fail to bring the gift of metaphysical healing if you follow the techniques presented to you in this chapter. If for one moment sickness or injury has colored your life drab and dark, you have spent too much time already in the grip of suffering. Begin now to bring a rainbow of color into your life by using the miracle of metaphysical healing to color your life and the lives of your loved ones perfectly healthy and happy.

COLORFUL SECRETS THAT WILL BRING YOU THE MIRACLE OF METAPHYSICAL HEALING

The secret properties of color presented to you here will touch your life in a way that it can never be the same. From this moment on you will be aware of the special place of color in fighting sickness and injury and bringing perfect health to replace all illness. Read these secrets carefully and know that they will be used by you to bring the glow of health to all you love.

1. The universal blueprint of redness which is present in all things colored red contains the secret of unlimited energy. It contains a special energy which brings the miracle of metaphysical healing in all cases of blood disease.

2. The universal blueprint of blueness present in all things

colored blue contains unlimited energy for bringing tranquility and peace. It also possesses unlimited energies for the destruction of all forms of infection.

3. The universal blueprint of greenness present in all things colored green contains unlimited energy for revitalizing the nervous system, the heart, and circulatory system.

4. The universal blueprint for orangeness present in all things colored orange contains unlimited energy for digestion and assimilation. This special energy also includes the assimilation of oxygen through the respiratory system. It is particularly useful in the treatment of asthma and all diseases involving the lungs and chest area.

5. The universal blueprint of yellowness present in all things colored yellow contains unlimited energy for purification. It is especially beneficial in bringing the miracle of metaphysical healing from diseases such as diabetes and those affecting the intestines and bowels.

6. The universal blueprint of indigoness is present in all things colored indigo and contains unlimited energy for the treatment of all illnesses and diseases affecting the area of the head, the eyes, the ears, and the nose. It also bears unlimited energy for the treatment of mental and emotional disorders.

7. The universal blueprint of violetness is present in all things colored violet and contains unlimited energy for regeneration of the nervous system. The energy associated with violetness is particularly effective in curing insomnia, mental disorders resulting from brain damage, physical illness and injury affecting the brain itself, and diseases and injuries to the eyes.

8. The universal blueprint of whiteness is present in all things colored white and contains unlimited energy for the treatment of all disease and all injury. The miraculous energy associated with this color heals the body and mind as a whole and is especially useful when a specific diagnosis of the individual's sickness or injury has not or cannot be made.

Now the miraculous secrets of the healing power of color are yours. From this day on you will be aware of the tremendous importance of color in your everyday life. Your mind and body are constantly absorbing the energies contained in the colors surrounding you, and with the use of your energized mind you can surround yourself with the essence of any color at will.

MOTHER USES MIRACULOUS COLOR TECHNIQUES TO STOP HER YOUNG SON'S ASTHMATIC ATTACKS

In a matter of minutes you will learn the actual miracle techniques that will allow you to use color in metaphysical healing to restore yourself and your loved ones to perfect health. Before you turn your attention to the metaphysical healing techniques that will allow you to color health into your daily life, I wish to share with you the story of Janet L. and her young son.

Janet L.'s young son was six years old when she first sought my help. Scotty was an attractive child with an unusually appealing smile for a six year old. As I look back on that first meeting I realize that the uniqueness of Scotty's smile was in part due to the fact that asthma had added a great deal of suffering to this child's life since he was three years old. That suffering showed through the innocent smile of a child too young to express it in words.

I learned from Janet that Scotty's attacks had grown more frequent and more severe since his fifth birthday. For 15 months Scotty had been suffering asthmatic attacks on an average of two and sometimes three attacks a day. Scotty had been to the best physicians and they had prescribed the newest and most effective medications available to them for the treatment of asthmatic attacks. The best in Scotty's case was not good enough, for the attacks continued to occur and Scotty continued to suffer.

"My son has suffered enough. I'm willing to do anything that will heal him and allow him to lead a normal life. Every time I watch him having an attack, see him gasping for air, my heart feels like it will burst. I want to help him so badly and yet I have felt so helpless."

Janet looked in Scotty's direction and a tear started to roll down her right cheek. He had seated himself in a large chair in a corner of the room and was intensely involved with a box of crayons and a Walt Disney coloring book.

"When I heard you on the radio talking about color and healing, it really struck a nerve with me. Scotty has always been sensitive to color ever since he was a baby. I just know that the color techniques of metaphysical healing can stop his asthmatic attacks. I want you to teach me how to use them for Scotty."

I gave Janet several sheets of paper explaining the universal blueprints of colors and the particular energies which each offers in the area of metaphysical healing. Since Scotty suffered from asthma, Janet was to use the universal blueprint for the color orange. I explained the step-by-step technique she was to follow in order to bring the miracle of metaphysical healing to her young son. Janet was to use this miraculous technique three times a day for one week and at the end of that time she was to telephone me and inform me of Scotty's progress. Janet thanked me and left in order to keep another appointment. She had promised to buy Scotty an ice cream soda on their way home and with Scotty's help she was not likely to forget that promise.

When one week had passed Janet called me to say that Scotty had gone six days without one asthmatic attack. In two weeks Scotty was to visit his physician for a periodic physical examination. "I'll let you know what happens during that visit. I can't wait to see Dr. N.'s face when he realizes that Scotty is cured of asthmatic attacks."

Janet was a woman of her word and two weeks later, immediately after leaving her doctor's office, she telephoned me. "I wish you could have been here to see the doctor's face. He's taking Scotty off his medication. It's been three weeks since Scotty has had an asthmatic attack and I know that that was the last one he will ever have.

"If you don't mind, Scotty and I will stop by to see you for a moment. Scotty has something he wants to give you."

An hour later Janet and Scotty were talking with me in person. Scotty's smile was still bright and attractive, but it had lost that unusual twist brought about by frequent and intensive physical suffering.

"My Mommy said you helped me to get well. I'm supposed to say thank you, and anyway I wanted to give you this myself."

Scotty handed me a large piece of paper, and when I looked at it I could not help but smile from ear to ear. He had ripped a page from his coloring book and presented me with the gift of the most beautiful orange duck I had ever seen.

The last time I heard from Janet L. was on Scotty's eighth birthday. She telephoned to say that Scotty was still free of asthmatic attacks and had even joined a peewee baseball team in his neighborhood. "Guess what? The uniforms they have are orange. How about that!"

The miraculous color techniques of metaphysical healing have opened up a whole new world of alternatives to Scotty L. Those same miracle techniques of metaphysical healing that allowed Scotty to be colored the picture of perfect health are available to you this very moment. Whether you use these miraculous techniques for yourself or for a loved one, they cannot fail to bring the miracle of metaphysical healing and a brighter, more colorful future to all whose life they touch.

YOUR MIRACLE TECHNIQUE THAT COLORS ASTHMATIC ATTACKS OUT OF YOUR LIFE

Repeat this miraculous technique three times a day. If you are using this miracle technique to restore a loved one to perfect health, insert your loved one's name in place of your own.

1. Select a location where you are not likely to be interrupted. Lie down or sit in a chair whose back is high enough to support your head.

2. Close your eyes and for a moment watch your intake and outflow of breath without attempting to control the process. Allow yourself to be aware of the relaxation which flows through your body and mind as you become more and more conscious of your own breathing.

3. Flood the screen of your mind's eye with a brilliant orange color. With your eyes still closed visualize everything around you colored a beautiful shade of bright orange. In your mind's eye see the air itself bearing a beautiful orange color.

Take a deep breath and, as you inhale, visualize or imagine pulling in long streams of orange colored light. Let your consciousness follow the inflow of this orange color through your nasal passages and into your lungs. Allow your consciousness to follow this orange light throughout your body and be very aware of the relaxation which overtakes both your body and mind. Repeat this breathing exercise three times, each time pulling in bright orange light and following that light through the use of your mind's eye throughout your entire body.

4. Through the power of your energized mind, repeat the following words to yourself mentally: "Through the miraculous force of my energized mind and the supreme intelligence of my high self, I will that the universal blueprint of orangeness bearing all the unlimited strength which it contains to be focused

immediately throughout my respiratory system. I will that the unlimited energy possessed by the universal blueprint of orangeness be released into my body and mind, freeing me from all asthmatic attacks and respiratory illnesses, and returning me from this point forward to perfect and unmarred physical and mental health.''

5. Again take a deep breath through your nose and visualize the inflow of orange light into your body and mind. Allow the universal blueprint of orangeness to concentrate its presence and strength throughout your respiratory system and watch this process by creating a mental motion picture of its progress on the mental screen of your own energized mind. Repeat this breathing exercise three times. With each new breath be aware of the added strength and vitality which is introduced to your system by the presence of the universal blueprint of orangeness.

6. Be aware once again of the intake and outflow of your own breathing without any attempt to control the process. Allow your mind to be totally aware of the complete relaxation which flows through your body, calming and dispelling its tensions and flowing into your mind with the same peace and tranquility.

7. Repeat the following words to yourself mentally: ''Through the miraculous power of energized mind and the unlimited energies released throughout my body by the universal blueprint of orangeness, I am free of all asthmatic attacks. Asthmatic attacks will no longer interrupt my body's natural desire to be 100 percent healthy. With the force of my energized mind I will that my body and mind shall impel itself totally and constantly in the direction of perfect health.''

8. Open your eyes and go about your daily life.

This miraculous color technique will bring the miracle of metaphysical healing and free you and your loved ones from the pain and horror of asthmatic attacks. You will find your life filled with sunshine and the bright colors of perfect health.

COLORS YOU SHOULD AVOID IN CERTAIN SITUATIONS

It is a fact that all colors are neither good nor bad, but simply possess and radiate certain energies. You will find it desirable to avoid certain of these energies when specific situations in your life are such that their presence would aggravate instead of heal. In line with this fact you will find that the choice of certain colors of clothing are best avoided in certain situations.

1. Red is not a good choice of color for clothing or surroundings for any individual who is emotionally upset, hysterical, or extremely overtired. The vital energies present in the universal blueprint of redness can, in these situations, overload an individual with too much energy and make sought-after tranquility more difficult to achieve.

2. Gray is to be avoided in clothing and in surroundings by any individual feeling emotionally depressed. In situations where an individual has allowed himself to give in to negativism concerning health or a situation of life, gray should also be avoided.

3. Blue should be avoided by all individuals who find themselves depleted in physical or mental energies. When the physical, emotional, or mental energy levels are low, blue in clothing or surroundings should be avoided. The unlimited tranquilizing energies of the universal blueprint of blueness would not have a beneficial effect in increasing energy levels, but rather would add to the low ebb of energy felt by the individual.

You have already gained a knowledge of colors that will allow you to make the proper decision as to when a specific color should be avoided. You will find this simple yet beneficial procedure will add immeasurably in touching your life with a healthy glow that will radiate to the lives of your loved ones.

COLOR CAN BRING CALM WHEN CONDITIONS CALL OUT CHAOS

Have you ever stood in the midst of a family crisis wishing there were something you could do to restore calmness to your loved ones? Whether that calmness was lost through physical pain, physical separation, or tragic accident, standing around feeling helpless is not a pleasant circumstance in which to find yourself. You and all who read this book need never stand helpless again in the face of any emergency. With the knowledge presented to you concerning the miracle of metaphysical healing, you can free yourself and your

loved ones from physical pain, restore health to diseased bodies, and
you can also bring tranquility to a mind seething with grief or panic.

You have the power to use the miracle of metaphysical healing
and the miraculous color techniques presented to you here to bring
peace to the most chaotic situation. You will not need tranquilizers or
any drug in order to bring about this peace, you will need only the
knowledge you gain in this chapter that will allow you to use the
miraculous color techniques to soothe your own mind and heart and
those of your loved ones.

YOUR MIRACLE COLOR TECHNIQUE FOR THE TREATMENT OF EMOTIONAL UPSETS

You may use this miracle technique in both crisis situations and
in circumstances where emotional upset is long-standing. In the
situation where a crisis exists you will find that following the step-
by-step method for the introduction of calmness and tranquility will
bring peace to the person or individuals to whom the miraculous color
technique is directed.

In situations of long-standing emotional upsets this miraculous
color technique should be followed three times a day. You will
quickly find that peace and calmness has replaced all mental and
emotional upset in your own life or the life of the loved one for whom
you are using the miracle of metaphysical healing.

1. Choose a location where you are not likely to be interrupted.
Either lie down or sit in a chair whose back is high enough to
support your head.

2. Close your eyes and for a moment be totally aware of your
intake and outflow of breath without making any attempt to
control this process. Allow yourself to be aware of the total
calmness which begins to flow through your entire body and
mind.

3. Allow the mental screen of your inner mind to be totally
covered with the universal blueprint of blueness. Allow this
blueness to fill every corner of your mind, bringing peace and
tranquility wherever it touches.

Without opening your eyes imagine or visualize everything
in your world permeated by the universal blueprint of blueness.

Visualize the air itself colored a beautiful shade of dark, peaceful blue.

4   As you take a deep breath through your nostrils, imagine or visualize that you are pulling blue light into yourself and that this blue light is circulating throughout your entire body innovating and calming your entire nervous system and mind. Repeat this exercise three times, allowing yourself to be totally aware of the complete calmness in your mind and body as your mind's eye is conscious of the universal blueprint of blueness flowing throughout your entire nervous system and filling your mind completely.

5. Repeat the following words to yourself mentally: "As the universal blueprint of blueness flows into my body, I am aware of its journey throughout my entire nervous system. I am completely conscious of the fact that it is filling my mind, adding calmness and strength in place of emotional agitation and disquiet. With the passage of the universal blueprint of blueness through my mind and body I am experiencing a peace deeper than any I have known before and a calmness which no outside circumstances can disturb. I am totally at peace within myself and am in harmony with all of nature."

6. Again take a deep breath through your nostrils bringing the universal blueprint of blueness into your body by inhaling blueness itself. Allow yourself to be even more aware of the calmness spreading throughout your body and mind as you follow the journey of blueness throughout your nervous system. Repeat this exercise three times. With each repetition be more and more aware of the calmness which flows throughout your body and within your mind.

7. For a moment watch your breath without any attempt to control it. Be completely aware of how attuned you feel to all of nature and to your own natural inclination toward perfect health of body and mind.

8. Open your eyes and go about your daily life.

This fantastic color technique allows you to bring peace and tranquility into the most chaotic situations. With the secrets of the miracle of metaphysical healing you are truly a peacemaker, for you bring peace not only externally but introduce tranquility into the hearts and minds of all you love. The miracle of metaphysical healing and the miraculous color technique you have just learned allows you to give the most precious gift one person can offer to another, the priceless gift of inner peace.

WOMAN USES MIRACULOUS COLOR TECHNIQUE TO INCREASE HER OWN ENERGY LEVEL

How many times have you spoken the words, or heard them spoken by someone else, "I wish I had more energy"? You, like millions of other people, have most likely found yourself in a situation at some time in your life when an increase in your energy level would have been of great benefit to you. You may have thought that there was nothing you could do to change your own energy level and that some people just had more energy than others. While it is true that some individuals do exhibit a higher energy level than others, it is not true that you are a victim of whatever energy level you possess. You have the ability to increase your energy a hundredfold, a thousandfold, and upward into regions where numbers grow into insignificance.

Whenever I meet an individual who talks about his or her lack of energy and the helplessness to do anything about it, I am reminded of Martha B. When I first met Martha she asked with sincere puzzlement written across her face, "Where do you get all the energy to be involved in so many things?" Before I had a chance to answer her question, Martha B. went on to explain that she had felt an emptiness in her life for many years because she was not able to take part in all the activities in which she shared an interest. Martha had been married to a man for nine years who, in addition to being one of the leading businessmen in their city, was very involved in participator sports. Ron B. was an excellent tennis player, golfer, and had recently completed a course in scuba diving and was pursuing this new interest with a great deal of enthusiasm.

"It seems that the more Ron does, the more energy he has to do other things. I really wish I could keep up with him. I'm interested in all the sports he likes, but I just don't have the energy it takes to pursue any of them."

As the conversation continued I explained to Martha that every individual has at his or her disposal an infinite amount of energy. The only thing that stands between a low and high energy level is a person's knowledge of how to get in touch with the source of infinite energy available to him. If anyone sincerely wanted to change his energy level, it could be done by following a simple, yet miraculous, technique of metaphysical healing involving the use of color. Martha sincerely wanted to change her energy level and so we discussed the exact steps she was to follow in order to release the infinite energy within her.

It was three weeks before I heard from Martha again. She called me long distance from the Bahamas to inform me that she and Ron were scuba diving and having a wonderful time.

"This is just great! I feel like a completely new woman—and, believe me, Ron really likes the change.

"We've been here for two days now and we plan to stay for an entire week. I had to teach Ron the metaphysical healing technique you taught me. For a change he was having trouble keeping up with my energy level.

"Do you realize this miracle color technique could put vitamin companies out of business? I never had so much energy in all my life and believe me it's a lot of fun being able to do the things I've always wanted to take part in."

Martha talked for about 15 minutes and finally closed with the remark, "It's a good thing my energy level is so high. I have a feeling I'm going to need that extra strength when I get the phone bill for this call."

Martha has been accompanying Ron on many of his business trips and if I were a stamp collector I'd be in an enviable position since post cards from the couple have come from many different countries. The infinite energy source available to every human being has enriched Martha B.'s life beyond words. What better way to say thank you for the gift of life than to live it fully?

You now have the opportunity to contact this infinite energy source within yourself through the miracle of metaphysical healing and the use of miraculous color techniques. Regardless of what your energy level has been in the past, know now that you can have an infinite amount of energy available to you simply by following the failproof technique presented to you in this chapter. You need never worry again about a lack of energy. Learn this technique now and you will always have the energy needed to achieve whatever goal you set and to accomplish whatever task you undertake.

YOUR MIRACLE COLOR TECHNIQUE FOR BECOMING A HUMAN DYNAMO

Perform this miraculous technique three times a day until you notice the drastic change which will take place in your energy level. When your energy level has increased to your satisfaction, perform this miracle exercise once a day in order to maintain contact with your infinite energy source.

1. Select a location in which you are not likely to be interrupted. Lie down or sit in a chair whose back is high enough to support your head.

2. Close your eyes and for a moment let your consciousness be aware of your own intake and outflow of breath without any attempt to control the process.

3. Allow your consciousness to be flooded with the color red. The universal blueprint for redness will radiate its infinite energy throughout your awareness.

     With the eye of your inner mind follow the universal blueprint of redness as it fills your mind and your body.

4. Take a deep breath through your nostrils and visualize yourself inhaling redness itself. Relax your stomach muscles immediately and allow your consciousness to follow the color red as it fills every area of your body and mind. Repeat this process three times and with each intake of breath be aware of the increased energy which is made available to you.

5. Repeat the following words to yourself mentally: "Through the use of my energized mind I am able to take full advantage of the limitless energy which the universal blueprint of redness makes available to me. My mind and body are flooded with infinite energy and all tiredness and fatigue have left me and been replaced with an inexhaustible supply of pure energy. My high self, through the power of my energized mind, will keep me in constant touch with my own source of infinite power."

6. Again take a deep breath, extending the diaphragm, and visualize yourself inhaling the universal blueprint of redness. Relax your stomach muscles completely and allow your consciousness to follow the path of redness throughout your entire mind and body as it makes available to each of your cells an

infinite amount of energy. Repeat this process three times, and with each repetition allow yourself to be more aware of the inexhaustible source of power made available to you.

7. Allow your consciousness to be totally aware of your own breathing process. Make no attempt to control the intake and outflow of breath, but only watch your breathing through the eyes of your consciousness.

Allow yourself to be aware of the new energy which flows through you and the infinite source of energy which stands ready to serve you at will.

8. Open your eyes and go about your daily life.

This miraculous color technique will bring the miracle of metaphysical healing to all who suffer from an inadequate supply of energy. You and your loved ones need never hesitate at participating at any activity because of a lack of energy. With this miraculous color technique you now have available to you an inexhaustible source of energy and an infinite source of power. Follow this miraculous technique faithfully and you will never know fatigue again.

six

The Miracle of Metaphysical Healing Can Cure Strongly Resistant Illness

Even the toughest illness can be cured through the miracle of metaphysical healing. There are many diseases today which the majority of people in our world consider too tough for traditional medicine to handle. Because of their resistance to cures offered through medical science, many of these diseases are considered virtually incurable. The miracle of metaphysical healing is a most powerful weapon in the fight against the "tough" or virtually "incurable" illness.

You, like millions of other people, have undoubtedly been exposed to the negative and illness-producing brainwashing that is presented in books, movies, and on television. What reader could truthfully say that he or she has never listened to a story or read a book whose plot centered around the death of one of the main characters because that individual had contracted a deadly and virtually "incurable" disease? It is unfortunate that such sickness-producing brainwashing is presented to us in a form of entertainment with little or no thought as to the effect it has on the lives of those who are exposed to its negativity. It would be interesting and yet extremely sad to know the actual number of people who have contracted dreaded illnesses after having the illness presented to them through the mass media.

The faculties of medical schools are quite aware that a great number of medical students are "sitting ducks" for what is known as "the medical student's syndrome." This label is an attempt to identify the process by which young medical students studying the particular symptoms of a specific disease become convinced that they themselves have contracted this illness and actually begin to exhibit the symptoms of the disease. When the young student is cured of the idea that he is a victim of the specific disease, the symptoms and pain associated with that disease are also cured. This is an example of the infinite power of man's mind in producing and curing illness presented to us from medical schools around the world where this phenomena is well-known.

If a man or woman is convinced that he or she will become ill, those thought patterns will often be brought into actuality and illness will actually strike the individual. If an individual is convinced that the disease afflicting his body is strongly resistant to cure and the physicians treating that individual are also convinced that the disease is strongly resistant to cure, there is little chance that a cure will be found quickly and without much suffering to the individual. When the label "strongly resistant" is placed on any sickness or disease, it is a statement that conventional medicine knows no quick or easy cures for that disease. When the label "strongly resistant" is accepted by the patient for any disease from which he suffers, it is a statement that the patient has given up all hope of a quick cure and has sentenced himself to long-term suffering and perhaps even death. The instrument by which death is caused in such cases is not the disease afflicting the patient, but the negative and malignant belief that a cure for this disease will be a long time in coming and that the disease may even end in death. This fallacious belief that there is little chance for a cure for the strongly resistant disease combined with the abandonment of the hope for recovery is the definition of the word "incurable" as it is used in this book.

Once the individual gives up, abandons hope, and professes a belief that no cure is possible, the individual is truly beaten by the illness. It is important to realize that the individual can be beaten by his or her own negative thinking and ignorance concerning the infinite power of energized mind to bring the miracle of metaphysical healing to even the toughest and most resistant of diseases.

You already know that you have within you the power to use the miraculous techniques presented to you in this book to bring the gift of metaphysical healing to yourself and your loved ones. In this chapter you will be made aware of the fact that the miracle of metaphysical healing can bring a cure to even the most resistant illness. Too often negative thinking and an ignorance of one's own ability creates the circumstance which too often passes as an "incurable" illness. With the knowledge already presented to you in this book, the miraculous techniques for metaphysical healing which you will learn in this chapter, you can bring the gift of perfect health to yourself and your loved ones who may be said to be suffering from a strongly resistant illness.

THROUGH METAPHYSICAL HEALING I AM CURED OF WHAT MANY CONSIDERED INCURABLE

The American Indians have a saying that goes, "Don't judge a man until you walk a mile in his moccasins." That saying was shouted to me by a young man suffering from paralysis who also said, "What right do you have to tell people to be hopeful or think positively? How do you know what it's like to be told there is no known cure for your paralysis or some other disease that has knocked your feet out from under you? If you've never been there, lady, you can't really know what it's like to have that kind of sentence pronounced on you."

This young man, John L., may have had a very good point, but in this case he was way off-base. (Later in this chapter this young man's situation will be discussed in detail.) I knew then and I know now what it's like to be told that a paralyzed limb will never move again. Eleven medical specialists ranging from general practitioners to neurosurgeons told me that the paralysis in my right arm could not be cured. That sentence was pronounced almost eight years ago and today I have the full use of my right arm.

The fact that that was not the first time I had heard such a sentence pronounced did not make the message any easier to live with. In 1961 I was involved in an accident in which I sustained a serious head injury. As a result of that injury I experienced the gradual loss of my eyesight, like two gigantic swinging doors moving closed to block out my view of the world. Thirteen doctors said that my blindness would be permanent and they all agreed that the pinhole of vision left to me was something for which I should be very grateful, but not count on keeping. My view of the world changed drastically as blindness claimed my eyesight. If you wish to see the world through my eyes at that time, stick a straight pin through a piece of paper, withdraw it and look through the hole left by that pin. If you haven't guessed by now, it leaves a lot to be desired.

You will most likely agree with me that one "incurable" sentence is enough for anyone and two "incurable" sentences are more than enough for anyone. As it turned out I was to have three "incurable" sentences in all. The same head injury which had produced the diagnosis of blindness and the prognosis of incurable was the first such sentence. Paralysis of my right arm with a diagnosis confirming that paralysis and a prognosis of incurable was the third sentence I was to receive in the "incurable" category. Sandwiched in between those two sentences came the diagnosis of epilepsy—the result of the same injury that had claimed my eyesight, and a prognosis of incurable. If you think I turned immediately to the miracle of metaphysical healing, you are 100 percent wrong. I was a very angry young woman and as much as it pains me to admit it, I wasted more than nine years venting my anger on myself, people around me, and even God. If it had been at all possible, I know I would have punched God right in the nose, and it only made me more angry to think that I'd have to use my left hand to do it. That's quite an admission if you consider the fact that prior to this accident I had spent almost two years of my life as a cloistered nun.

Somehow everything I had learned as a child concerning the miracle of metaphysical healing and everything I had read in the Scriptures concerning the keys that unlock this miraculous secret was all forgotten by me. I didn't know the true meaning of the word incurable and so when doctors said that the injuries from which I suffered were all permanent, I threw away all hope and in complete ignorance I filled myself with hostility and resentments. What I had known in my head all my life concerning a human being's own power through the force of his mind to bring healing to illness or injury had never been learned by heart. It seems that what is learned only intellectually and not by heart can be easily shouted down by a critic or a well-intentioned physician who diagnoses an illness or injury and states that you have little or no chance of recovery.

Perhaps I got tired of being angry or maybe the information that had filled my head for years had finally made it to my heart, maybe it was the grace of God, or a combination of all three, but I finally decided that I would be cured of blindness, of epilepsy, and of paralysis. I told my plan to two friends and they offered to perform the exercise with me on my behalf. We used the same techniques which are presented for you in this book and in ten days I had been entirely cured through the miracle of metaphysical healing and enjoyed then, as I do now, the blessing of perfect health.

I am grateful for the health that I enjoy and I want every man, woman, and child to share the same wonderful gift. It is for this reason that this book has been written, in order to share with you the miraculous techniques which bring the blessing of the miracle of metaphysical healing to all those who will follow the foolproof techniques that will bring perfect health in the face of illness and make that illness a thing of the past. You will not have to wait as I did because these miraculous techniques are at your fingertips at this very moment. I sincerely believe that one of the reasons it took me so long to decide to use the miracle of metaphysical healing was that I might be impressed with the value of these miraculous techniques and share them with the world. You at this very moment are taking part in that sharing.

Now you will learn the miraculous techniques which brought the miracle of metaphysical healing to me when physicians said that healing in my case was out of the question. Those same physicians were surprised, yet happy, for me when I was examined after the miracle of metaphysical healing had returned me to perfect health. Keep in mind that an examination by a physician in order to document that an actual cure has taken place is not to be overlooked. The miracle of metaphysical healing works alongside of conventional medicine and never should be thought of as something which attempts to discredit or do away with traditional medical practices. Metaphysical healing is meant to be an enrichment for the medical profession, an additional tool which every individual may use for his or her own well-being.

YOUR VIDEO-MEDIC TECHNIQUE FOR THE CURE OF PARALYSIS

The miraculous technique which follows worked for me and countless other individuals in restoring freedom of movement to paralyzed limbs. It will also work for you and all your loved ones.

Perform this miraculous exercise three times a day and you will find that the miracle of metaphysical healing will soon bring perfect health and freedom of movement to you and all for whom you perform this failproof exercise.

1. Select a location where you are not likely to be disturbed. Lie down or sit in a chair whose back is high enough to support your head.

2. Close your eyes and for a moment let your consciousness be aware of your own intake and outflow of breath without attempting to control the breathing process. Be aware of the relaxation which flows through your body as you turn your consciousness to your own breathing process.

3. Take a deep breath through your nostrils, extending your diaphragm, and immediately following inhalation, relax your stomach muscles completely. Allow your consciousness to follow the flow of oxygen through your body and allow its journey to terminate in the area of your head. Repeat this exercise three times and with each repetition allow yourself to be more and more aware of the relaxation which fills both your body and mind.

4. Repeat the following words to yourself mentally: "Through the power of energized mind new and healthy cells are replacing all damaged cells within my body. Limbs that were once restricted in movement are now completely healed and can move freely. The miracle of metaphysical healing through the power of my energized mind has restored or replaced all paralyzed cells within my body and brought me the blessing of perfect health and unrestricted movement."

5. On the screen of your own inner consciousness create your own mental motion picture. See yourself clearly with any previously paralyzed portion of your body moving freely.

Now add sound to your mental motion picture and hear specific friends and relatives saying things to express their astonishment at your complete recovery through the miracle of metaphysical healing. For example, "How in the world did you ever get the use of your arm back? I know your doctors said it would never happen. I'm really glad for you; it's wonderful to see you completely healthy again."

6. Now create your own mental motion picture in which you will visit your physician and your doctor will express astonishment at your complete recovery from paralysis. Add the miracle of sound to your mental motion picture and hear your doctor speak the following words, "I didn't think I'd ever see the day when you'd be able to use that paralyzed arm again. (Mentally insert the proper words which will describe new freedom of movement to the portion of your body which is paralyzed.) I don't know how it happened, but I'm very glad for you."

"Thank you, doctor, I'm awfully happy myself. I'm very thankful that I have the full use of my arm again."

7. Again take a deep breath through your nostrils, extending your diaphragm. Completely relax your stomach muscles when you have completed your inhalation and allow your consciousness to follow your breath throughout your body, bringing it to rest in the area of your head. Repeat this exercise three times, each time allowing yourself to be more and more aware of the increased relaxation which flows through your mind and body.

8. Allow your consciousness to be totally aware of your breathing process without any attempt to control it. Again be conscious of the relaxation which continues to flow throughout your mind and body.

9. Open your eyes and go about your daily life.

This miraculous video-medic technique is guaranteed to bring the miracle of metaphysical healing to all paralyzed areas of your body. It cannot fail to work for you just as it worked for me and countless others in restoring freedom of movement to previously paralyzed bodies

Don't waste another moment of your life in unnecessary restriction and suffering. Begin today to use the miracle of metaphysical healing through your miraculous video-medic technique in order to bring the blessing of perfect health to yourself and your loved ones.

YOUR VIDEO-MEDIC TECHNIQUE FOR THE CURE OF EPILEPSY

Before the miracle of metaphysical healing cured me of epilepsy, I was experiencing on an average of ten to 12 seizures a day. In an attempt to control my epileptic seizures physicians had prescribed dilantin and phenobarbital which I took three times a day. It was these medications which reduced the number of epileptic seizures I experienced daily.

Without these medications my seizures were so numerous each day that it would have been ridiculous to try to keep an accurate record of their numbers.

The miraculous video-medic technique which follows is the exact method which worked for me and countless others in bringing a complete cure from epilepsy through the miracle of metaphysical healing. Perform this miraculous exercise faithfully and it cannot fail to bring the miracle of metaphysical healing to you and your loved ones who suffer from epilepsy.

Read the exercise through completely at least once before following this miraculous technique. Perform the video-medic technique at least three times a day and you will soon find that the gift of perfect health has been given to you or any loved one for whom this exercise is performed.

1. Select a location in which you are not likely to be disturbed. Lie down or sit in a chair whose back is high enough to support your head.

2. Close your eyes and for a moment let your consciousness be totally aware of your breathing process without any attempt to control it. As your mind's eye watches your intake and outflow of breath, be totally aware of the complete relaxation which begins to flow through your body and mind.

3. Take a deep breath through your nostrils and immediately after inhalation completely relax your stomach muscles. Allow your consciousness to follow the path of that breath through your entire body and bring it to rest in the area of your head. Repeat this exercise three times and with each repetition be more and more aware of the increased relaxation which completely fills your body and mind.

4. Repeat the following words to yourself mentally: "Through the actions of my high self and the infinite power of my energized mind I will that I am cured of all epilepsy and epileptic seizures. I will that the miracle of metaphysical healing bring new strength and the gift of perfect health to my body and mind. Since I have received the blessing of metaphysical healing and the gift of perfect health I will no longer suffer from epileptic seizures, nor will I be epileptic."

5. Use the power of your energized mind to create your own mental motion picture. See yourself in the presence of your loved ones and add to this the miracle of sound. Hear your loved ones speaking words such as, "We are so glad that you are no longer epileptic. I know we can't be quite as happy as you are, but believe me we're overjoyed that you no longer suffer from epileptic seizures."

"Thank you for sharing in my happiness. You're right, it's wonderful not to be epileptic any more."

6. Continue your mental motion picture and create a scene that will place you in your doctor's office. Add the miracle of sound to your mental motion picture and hear your doctor speak the following words, "I'm happy to tell you that you no longer have epilepsy. All the tests confirm that you are completely cured of epilepsy and epileptic seizures. We can begin today to withdraw you from all medications for epilepsy. This gradual reduction in the amount of medication you take will go on for about a month before you need take no medication at all. You see your body gets used to dilantin and phenobarbital and if we took you off the medication suddenly with no reduction period, it might throw you into a grand mal seizure.

"Believe me you have nothing to worry about; you are completely cured of epilepsy. I don't know how it happened, but I am happy for you."

"Thank you very much, doctor. I'll follow your instructions for the gradual reduction in medication and I'll look forward to the day when I will not have to take any medications at all. A month or so does not seem very long to wait for that day after all this time of daily epileptic seizures. I'm awfully happy that I am no longer an epileptic."

7. Again take a deep breath through your nostrils, extending the diaphragm as you inhale, and completely relaxing your stomach muscles once you have completed your inhalation. Allow your consciousness to follow that breath throughout your body and bring it to rest finally in the area of your head. Repeat this breathing exercise three times and with each repetition allow your consciousness to be more and more aware of the complete relaxation which fills your body and mind.

8. For a brief moment watch your breathing process without any attempt to control it. Again allow your consciousness to be aware of the complete relaxation which exists within your body and mind.

9. Open your eyes and go about your daily life.

This miraculous video-medic technique is guaranteed to bring the blessing of perfect health to you and any of your loved ones who suffer from epilepsy. Begin today to use this miracle technique so that you and your loved ones will not have to suffer another day, but can begin enjoying the gift of complete and perfect health.

Do not allow yourself to lose sight of the fact that a visit to your physician is of extreme importance once you have received your cure from epilepsy. You will need your doctor's direction in the documentation of your cure and in the gradual reduction of the amount of medication given for the control of your epileptic seizures. Your physician is the best judge concerning your withdrawal from medication since the human body itself develops a certain dependency upon drugs given for the control of epilepsy.

Begin using your miracle video-medic technique today so that a visit to your physician will come even more quickly. This miraculous technique cannot fail to cure you and anyone for whom it is performed from epilepsy and epileptic seizures if you but follow it faithfully as outlined for you.

YOUR MIRACULOUS VIDEO-MEDIC TECHNIQUE
FOR THE CURE OF BLINDNESS

Naturally you are aware of the fact that if a person is blind, he or she will not be able to read the steps of this exercise for himself. With this fact in mind it is taken for granted that someone reading this exercise will be using the technique in order to bring the blessing of metaphysical healing to a loved one, or that the person reading this technique has enough eyesight left so that no matter how difficult it might be, he or she is able to struggle through the reading of the exercise on their own. It is hoped that one day this entire book will be available on records, eight track tapes, and cassettes.

The miraculous video-medic technique presented below is the exact method I followed in order to bring the miracle of metaphysical healing to myself and receive a complete cure from blindness. Do not allow its simplicity to fool you for within these steps is the key to unlocking the infinite power available to you in your energized mind in order that you, too, may bring the gift of metaphysical healing to yourself or a loved one who suffers from blindness.

Repeat this miraculous technique three times a day. As with all the miraculous methods included in this book, if you are performing this technique for a loved one you only need insert the proper pronoun and name wherever common sense indicates that it is appropriate.

1. Select a location where you are not likely to be disturbed. Lie down or sit in a chair whose back is high enough to support your head.

2. Close your eyes and for a moment give your full attention to your own breathing process without making any attempt to control this process. Allow yourself to be aware of the complete relaxation which begins to flood your body and mind.

3. Take a deep breath through your nostrils, extending the diaphragm as you inhale, and relaxing your stomach muscles completely at the completion of your inhalation. Allow your consciousness to follow the path of the oxygen which you have inhaled throughout your body bringing it to rest finally in the area of your head. Repeat this process three times and with each inhalation allow yourself to be more and more aware of the total relaxation which floods your mind and body.

4. Repeat the following words to yourself mentally: "Through the limitless power of my energized mind and the total wisdom of my high self all energy within and without my own being is in motion to return the gift of eyesight to me. All damaged cells in my body are at this time repaired, restored, or replaced so that in spite of whatever damage has existed it is now healed and the gift of eyesight is returned to me through the miracle of metaphysical healing."

5. In your inner consciousness create your own mental motion picture. In your mind's eye see yourself actually seeing. See yourself looking around and filling your eyes with sights you have never seen or have not seen in a very long time.

   Now add the miracle of sound to your mental motion picture and hear your loved ones say the following or similar words to you: "It really is a miracle that you can see. I would never have believed it possible, but who can argue with facts? You are seeing and that is wonderful. I'm really happy for you, but I know no matter how happy I am it cannot compare with how you must feel within yourself."

   "Thank you for sharing my happiness. You're right, it is wonderful to be able to see."

6. Create your own mental motion picture of a visit to your physician. See yourself being examined by your doctor and hear the following or a similar conversation take place between you.

"I don't understand how it's possible, but I cannot argue with the fact that you are seeing. Medically I cannot explain it, but as a fellow human being I can tell you that I'm very happy for you."

"Thank you very much, doctor. I knew that in addition to being interested in my healing itself, you would also share in my happiness at being able to see."

7. Take a deep breath through your nostrils and extend your diaphragm as you inhale. As you complete your inhalation completely relax your stomach muscles and allow your consciousness to follow the passage of your inhaled breath throughout your body finally coming to rest in the area of your head. Repeat this process three times, each time allowing yourself to be more and more aware of the deep relaxation which is now present in your entire body and mind.

8. For a moment watch your breathing without any attempt to control the process. Continue to be aware of the deep relaxation flooding your mind and body and enjoy the sensation of being completely at rest.

9. Open your eyes and go about your daily life.

Readers who have always enjoyed the gift of eyesight may be surprised to read instructions directing the closing and opening of the eyes in this exercise. There are many fallacies surrounding blindness and all of us would do well to keep in mind that a person suffering from blindness is no different from any human being except for the fact that his physical eyesight is not at that moment working.

With this video-medic technique you will find that the miracle of metaphysical healing is not long in coming, bringing its gift of eyesight to the person for whom this exercise is performed. Don't waste another moment. Begin using this technique today.

It goes without saying that I am extremely grateful for the miracle of metaphysical healing which has touched my own life. Now I wish to help all my fellow human beings use the miracle of metaphysical healing for themselves. You have within you a limitless source of power and your energized mind can bring the blessing of metaphysical healing to you today. Remember the definition of the word "incurable" used in this book, that the "incurable" disease is the resistant illness combined with your abandonment of all hope for a recovery. With this book and the techniques it places literally at your fingertips there is no reason for you or your loved ones to suffer illness, injury, or disease one minute longer. You have the miraculous power to bring metaphysical healing into your life and the lives of all you love. Begin to use that power now.

JOHN L. WAS TOO ANGRY TO ACCEPT ANYONE'S HELP, INCLUDING HIS OWN

Earlier in this chapter I told you that I would speak further concerning a young man suffering from paralysis and a severe case of anger and hostility. Nancy L., John's sister, brought him to me to learn about the miracle of metaphysical healing. John's right arm had been paralyzed for three years following an accident in which several nerves had been severed. He had come of his own free will and yet the anger and hostility which boiled inside him spilled over during our first meeting.

"It's easy for you and Nancy to talk—you both have the use of both your arms. No wonder you're not negative, you don't have anything to be negative about."

I must admit that as our conversation wore on and John's hostility did not let up, I became angry at the fact he was delaying his own healing through resentment and hostility. John's eyes opened wide and he looked shocked as my anger at the situation he was creating for himself was given expression. Nancy looked just as surprised as John as I shouted at him, "You hold on just a minute. You're not the only one who's ever suffered paralysis. I do know what I'm talking about. I've had a paralyzed right arm and I have the use of it today thanks to the miracle of metaphysical healing which, if you'd shut your mouth long enough to give me your attention, I'd be happy to share with you."

John's mouth and Nancy's, too, were opened just slightly in an attitude of pure shock, but not one word was uttered by either one of them. Their eyes looked as if they had doubled in size and as I realized their shock that I had shouted as I did, I had to fight hard not to laugh at their astonishment that I, too, was very human.

I told John what had happened in my own situation involving what medical doctors called "incurable" paralysis. He listened quietly as I explained the step-by-step technique I had used to bring the miracle of metaphysical healing to my own paralyzed right arm.

He and Nancy left, but not before John said, "It's sure worth a try. I have nothing to lose and a lot to gain."

Two weeks after that meeting I heard from Nancy L. and she told me that her brother John's arm had had its mobility completely restored. "The paralysis is completely gone. John is like a schoolboy on a long summer vacation. He really is happy."

Ten days after I heard from Nancy L., I received a post card from John L. The card expressed his thanks for the fact that I had shared with him the secret of metaphysical healing and conveyed his promise to share it with anyone he met who could also use the miracle of metaphysical healing. That was the last time I heard from John L., and when I ran into his sister six months ago she told me that John had moved to California and was doing very well in a new job. "The last time I saw John he told me no one would ever guess that his arm had ever been paralyzed."

John L. regained the use of his paralyzed arm by following the same video-medic technique presented to you earlier in this chapter. You, too, can bring the miracle of metaphysical healing to yourself and your loved ones who suffer from any form of paralysis.

WOMAN IS CURED OF KIDNEY DISEASE THROUGH THE MIRACLE OF ENERGIZED MIND

Did you happen to catch the TV show about two years ago with a plot that centered around five people who all needed an artificial kidney machine in order to go on living? The suspense in the TV drama was supposedly provided by the fact that only one of the five people could be placed on the machine and the remaining four would face certain death from a kidney disease known as polynephritis which had been given the prognosis of fatal and incurable. I found the TV movie pitiful for two reasons. The first thing that saddened me about the movie was the fact that anyone in this country should die not for lack of knowledge, but for lack of money. Even more sad was the fact that anyone suffering from this dreaded kidney disease should be pronounced incurable simply because medical science has not yet found a way in traditional medicine to bring about a cure. If the writer of that script had known about the miracle of metaphysical healing, he could have written an entirely different movie with completely different emotional overtones and a strikingly different ending.

Anyway, if you didn't see that particular movie I'm sure you've seen one with a plot very similar to it.

Patricia R. had seen that movie and many more like it before she learned that she herself was suffering from polynephritis. She didn't have to worry about whether she would be the lucky one to be chosen to be hooked up to an artificial kidney machine. There was no kidney machine available. If there had been ten artificial kidney machines available, this would not have made a big difference to Patricia R., for treatment on such machines was expensive and Patricia R. earned only $80 a week and had a savings account that amounted to $2100.

A close friend of Patricia's told her about the miracle of metaphysical healing and brought her to speak with me concerning metaphysical healing for the disease which now threatened her life. We talked for about an hour and Patricia finally said, "I'm not ready to give up and if ignorance is one big thing keeping me from getting in touch with such a miraculous power within myself, then teach me what I need to know in order to cure the 'incurable.' "

We went over the special miracle steps Patricia was to use in order to bring the gift of perfect health to herself and she left with a promise that she would keep in close touch. She phoned twice in the next month to tell me that she was feeling much better and during the second phone call she informed me that she had an appointment to see her urologist exactly one week from that day. Patricia promised that I would hear from her again after that examination.

When that phone call came from Patricia the news was all good. "I know it's been ten days instead of a week since I talked to you last, but I wanted to wait until all the reports were back from the doctor. It's gone. The polynephritis is gone. The doctor says I'm in excellent health and there's no evidence of disease of any kind in my body.

"He asked me if I had any idea what might have caused the cure so I told him exactly what I had been doing with the miracle of metaphysical healing. I don't know if he believed me or not—he looked awfully surprised—anyway, that's his problem. I am in 100 percent perfect health.

"Thank you so very much for sharing the miracle of energized mind with me."

As I said earlier, if the writer who wrote the script for that TV movie had only known about the miracle of metaphysical healing, the ending of his story would have been a very happy one and for many people just as surprising as any Alfred Hitchcock movie.

YOUR ENERGIZED MIND TECHNIQUE FOR THE MIRACULOUS CURE OF KIDNEY DISEASE

Repeat the following technique three times a day. It will bring the miracle of metaphysical healing to you or any loved one for whom you perform it.

1. Select a location where you are not likely to be disturbed. Lie down or sit in a chair with a back high enough to support your head.

2. Close your eyes and for a moment watch your breathing with no attempt to control it. Allow your consciousness to be very aware of the relaxation beginning to flow through your body and mind.

3. Take a deep breath through your nostrils, extending the diaphragm as you inhale, and completely relaxing your stomach muscles once inhalation is complete. Follow the passage of that breath through your body with your inner consciousness and bring it to rest finally in the area of your head. Repeat this exercise three times and with each repetition allow yourself to be more and more aware of the complete relaxation which is flowing through your body and mind.

4. Repeat the following words to yourself mentally: "Through the miracle of energized mind and at the direction of my high self I command that all cells within my kidneys and urinary tract which are damaged or diseased be restored or replaced immediately. I further command that my kidneys and urinary system be in complete harmony within itself and in total harmony with all other systems of my body."

5. Create your own mental motion picture and see yourself with your doctor. Add the miracle of sound and create a scene with the following plot. See your doctor clearly and hear him say the words, "My examination and test results indicate that you no longer suffer from a kidney disease. In fact, I can find no evidence of disease anywhere in your body. You are 100 percent in perfect health and we will discontinue all medication immediately."

"Thank you so much, Doctor, for everything you've done

for me. I'm sure I don't have to tell you how glad I am to hear that I no longer have any disease and that I am in perfect health.''

6. Take a deep breath through your nostrils, extending your diaphragm as you inhale. Completely relax your stomach muscles once you have completed your inhalation and allow your consciousness to follow the passage of your breath through your body, coming to rest finally in the area of your head. Repeat this process three times and with each repetition allow yourself to be more and more aware of the complete and total relaxation which floods your mind and body.

7. For a moment let your consciousness be aware of your breathing process without attempting to control it. Again be completely aware of the total and complete relaxation which now exists throughout your entire body and mind

8. Open your eyes and go about your daily life.

The aforementioned technique is a foolproof method which will bring the miracle of metaphysical healing to anyone suffering from kidney disease. If you or a loved one have been the victim of kidney disease, begin this exercise today. Do not spend another moment in physical or emotional anguish when the miracle of energized mind can so easily return you to perfect health.

YOUR MIRACULOUS METHOD OF ENERGIZED MIND FOR THE CURE OF INCURABLE DISEASE

The following failproof method for metaphysical healing is to be used with all incurable diseases not discussed individually in this chapter. Repeat this exercise three times a day and you will find that no disease, no matter how ominous its reputation, can withstand the miraculous power of your own energized mind in combination with this miraculous method.

1. Select a location in which you are not likely to be disturbed. Lie down or sit in a chair whose back is high enough to support your head.

2. Close your eyes and for a moment let your consciousness be focused completely on your intake and outflow of breath without making any attempt to control it. As you mentally watch

your own breathing process allow yourself to be aware of the relaxation which begins to flow through your body and mind.

3. Take a deep breath through your nostrils, extending your diaphragm as you inhale. Following inhalation of your breath, completely relax your stomach muscles and allow your consciousness to follow the breath through your body coming to rest finally in the area of your head. Repeat this process three times and with each repetition allow yourself to become more and more aware of the increased relaxation flooding your body and mind.

4. Repeat the following words to yourself mentally: "Through the power of my energized mind I stand in the wisdom of my high self and am aware of the fact that my body and mind are inclined naturally toward perfect health. I know with certainty that no disease is incurable since the power of my own energized mind is greater than any force upon this earth. I command that through the wisdom of my high self the power of my energized mind will be directed now to restore or replace all damaged or diseased cells within my body and return all my systems to a state of perfect and total well-being."

5. Create your own mental motion picture to which you will add the miracle of sound. See yourself with your loved ones and hear a discussion of the fact that you have been cured of all disease within your body.

Mentally see yourself in your doctor's office and hear your doctor state that according to his findings and test results all disease in your body is gone and you are in a state of perfect health.

6. Take a deep breath, extending your diaphragm as you inhale. Completely relax your stomach muscles on completion of your inhalation and allow your consciousness to follow your breath through your body, coming to rest in the area of your head. Repeat this process three times and with each repetition be more and more aware of the total and complete relaxation which is flooding your mind and body.

7. Repeat the following words to yourself mentally: "In spite of the fact that my conscious mind may be engaged in matters of daily living, my high self will continuously direct the power of my energized mind for the purpose of restoring me to complete

and total perfect health. The miracle of metaphysical healing through the power of my energized mind will be in continuous process within me so that once returned to a state of perfect health I shall maintain and enjoy that state always.''

8. Allow your consciousness to be aware of your intake and outflow of breath. Do not attempt to control your breathing process but be totally aware of the fact that complete and total relaxation now floods your mind and body.

9. Open your eyes and go about your daily life.

You are a most powerful human being. With the knowledge and miraculous techniques this book has placed at your disposal no illness, disease, or injury can withstand the power of your energized mind. You have had within you from the moment of your birth the miraculous ability to restore and maintain perfect health within yourself and your loved ones, and you now have the knowledge available to you to put that power to practical use. Because you now know the true meaning of the word ''incurable,'' you are now in a position to bring the miracle of metaphysical healing to yourself or any individual suffering from any disease, injury, or illness. You are truly a magnificent creation.

seven

The Miracle of Metaphysical Healing in Your Mental Medicine Cabinet

How many different medicines do you think there are in your medicine cabinet right now? Excluding prescription drugs for the moment, how many over-the-counter, non-prescription medicines would I find if I could open the door on your medicine chest right this moment? Without going to check, make an honest guess at the number of non-prescription medicines which you feel are present in the medicine cabinet of your own home.

If you have made your guess, leave this book for a moment and go to your medicine cabinet for an actual count. After you have made your honest tally come right back to this book.

How did your first estimate compare with the number of non-prescription drugs you actually found? In several instances did you find a number of bottles of the same medication? If your medicine cabinet is typical of medicine cabinets throughout our country, you found a generous variety of bottles, jars, and tubes.

The average stash of non-prescription medicines in the typical home today reflects the negative brainwashing to which we as human beings are exposed. It would be a better than a safe bet to say that you most likely found one or two headache remedies, a liquid and a tablet to combat nausea, a laxative in a liquid or tablet form, a liquid for the control of diarrhea, eye drops guaranteed to keep your eyes free of redness, perhaps a dozen tiny capsules guaranteed to relieve the symptoms of a cold, tiny tablets to control the symptoms of hay fever-like allergies, and nose drops for the special control of allergies affecting the nose. This is by no means a complete list of all the possible non-prescription remedies found in the average household today. It is, however, long enough to reflect the sad state in which many of our countrymen find themselves. It seems like a great majority of people expect to get sick and have such confidence in the fact that they will that they stockpile non-prescription drugs as ammunition in a war that is of their own making. The price of this self-declared war on an individual's health is devastating, and the financial cost is as shocking as the combined war debt of all countries involved in World War II.

With the information made available to you in this chapter you will not only enjoy perfect health, but you will cut your medical bills anywhere from 85 to 98 percent. Your remaining bill will depend on how frequently you find yourself in need of band-aids, mercuro-chrome, cotton balls, and Q-tips. In this situation time means not only money, but also health, so begin immediately to learn the contents of your mental medicine cabinet so that you may use the miracle of metaphysical healing in place of artificial remedies.

Every day hundreds of thousands of people take millions of aspirins to combat the pain of headaches which the mass media has told them every day they are sure to suffer. Almost all of the ads for these non-prescription headache remedies state that tension is the number one cause of the common headache. The cause of tension is the mental stress which individuals find themselves subjected to during their routine daily life.

You now have the opportunity to use the simple but miraculous technique presented here for the treatment of headaches and their causes. There will be no need for you to shop for this remedy and it will not cost you another cent since everything you need to use it effectively is already present within your mental medicine cabinet and the instructions given here for the miracle of metaphysical healing will tell you exactly how to use the abilities that are already yours.

YOUR MIRACLE TECHNIQUE FOR THE CURE OF HEADACHES

You may use this miraculous technique whenever you are the victim of a headache. It cannot fail to heal both your headache pain and the underlying mental stress which has brought it about.

1. Although it is not necessary, it is desirable that you can find a place where you can be alone for a few moments without

interruption. If this is not possible, situate yourself so that you may close your eyes for a few minutes in order to withdraw into your own consciousness.

2. Take a deep breath through your nostrils, extending the diaphragm as you inhale. Immediately relax your stomach muscles on the completion of your inhalation and allow your consciousness to follow the breath through your body, finally coming to rest in the area of your head. Repeat this process three times and with each repetition be more and more aware of the total relaxation spreading through your body and mind.

3. Repeat the following words to yourself mentally: "Through the wisdom of my high self and with the power of my energized mind I command that all unnecessary stress leave my body and mind immediately and that both my body and mind are now in a state of perfect health free of tension, stress, and pain. The wisdom of my high self and the power of my energized mind shall maintain me in this state of complete harmony."

4. Allow your consciousness to be aware of the intake and outflow of breath for a moment without any attempt to control the process. Allow yourself to be totally aware of the complete relaxation which is now flooding your body and mind.

5. Open your eyes and go about your daily life.

Do not allow yourself to be fooled by the apparent simplicity of this technique. This miraculous method packs more power for the relief of headache pain and mental stress than any headache remedy which money can buy. You need never suffer from headaches again since you now have the knowledge that will bring the miracle of metaphysical healing to your headache within a matter of moments.

A NERVOUS OR UPSET STOMACH CAN CAUSE A MULTITUDE OF PROBLEMS

Have you ever had an upset stomach ruin your day or evening? Whether your stomach upset is the result of nervous tension, overindulgence, or an intestinal bug, it can be cured very easily through the power of your energized mind. The miracle method of metaphysical healing involving five failproof steps is presented for you in this chapter and is guaranteed to bring tranquility to the most upset of stomachs. You need no longer wonder which non-prescription drug will work best for your upset stomach. You no longer need to spend money for bottles of pretty colored liquids or tablets that fizzle in a search for a remedy that will bring peace and harmony to a wildly churning stomach.

With the miraculous method presented below, no guesswork is necessary. Since it depends on the power of your energized mind for its success and since that power is limitless, this method cannot fail to heal even the sickest of sick stomachs. Learn this miraculous technique now and never waste another moment of your life suffering the miserable feeling that can accompany a nervous or upset stomach.

YOUR FIVE STEP MIRACLE METHOD FOR THE CURE OF A NERVOUS OR UPSET STOMACH

The miraculous method presented here may be used whenever you are disturbed by a nervous or upset stomach. It will never fail to bring relief and tranquility even in the most severe cases of nausea.

1. If at all possible find a location where you can be alone. If this cannot be accomplished easily, situate yourself in such a position that you may close your eyes for a few minutes and give your attention to your own consciousness.

2. Take a deep breath through your nostrils, extending the diaphragm as you inhale. On completion of your inhalation completely relax your stomach muscles and allow your awareness to follow the path of your breath throughout your body, coming to rest finally in the area of your head. Repeat this process three times, and with each repetition allow your consciousness to become more aware of the increased relaxation and tranquility flowing through your mind and body.

3. Repeat the following words to yourself mentally: "Through the wisdom of my high self and with the power of my energized mind I command that all tension, nausea, and upset leave my stomach and digestive track immediately. I command that the miracle of metaphysical healing shall immediately restore me to a state of perfect inner balance and that my high self with the power of my energized mind shall maintain me in that state."

4. For a brief moment allow your consciousness to be totally aware of the intake and outflow of your breath. Do not attempt

to control your breathing process, but allow yourself to be completely aware of the total tranquility and relaxation which now completely fills your body and mind.

5. Open your eyes and go about your daily life.

With this miracle method you will never be at the mercy of an upset stomach again. The miracle of metaphysical healing available to you in your mental medicine cabinet places you in complete control of your own physical and mental health. With the miracles available to you in your mental medicine cabinet you will be able to enjoy and maintain the health which you were created to experience.

CONVENTIONAL MEDICINE KNOWS NO CURE FOR THE COMMON COLD

Have you ever heard it said that conventional medicine can cure pneumonia, but can do nothing to cure the common cold? This one fact has been the scene for many a cartoon and comedy situation. In real life, however, the individual suffering from that common cold rarely finds the cold very funny. The stuffy head, rasping cough, watery eyes, muscle aches, sore throat, and fever that accompany many colds can, if allowed to do so, make an individual's life pretty miserable. Each year millions of individuals who have allowed themselves to be overcome by the common cold spend millions of dollars on remedies that promise to alleviate cold symptoms, but are clearly not offering a cure for the common cold. You, as a reader of this book, need never be in that category again. You need never suffer the discomfort of a cold if you use the miracle techniques presented for your benefit in earlier chapters that will allow you to maintain your state of perfect health. If, through some laxity on your part, a cold does happen to come your way, the longest period you will have to endure it is one hour if you use the miracle of metaphysical healing in the miraculous technique for the cure of the common cold presented in this chapter. Why should you waste your time feeling miserable with a cold when in an hour or less you can be completely cured of that cold and feeling in tiptop condition? Who would be so foolish as not to learn this miraculous technique which takes only a few moments of your time and can save you weeks of unnecessary suffering?

You have the power to cure the common cold and it is now up to you to learn to use that power for yourself and your loved ones. Follow the miraculous technique presented for you below and say good-by to cold miseries and expensive bills for cold remedies ranging from nose sprays, candy flavored cough syrup, and eight- and 12-hour congestion relievers.

YOUR MIRACULOUS ENERGIZED MIND TECHNIQUE FOR THE CURE OF THE COMMON COLD

Use this miracle technique at the first onset of cold symptoms. The time you allow to elapse between the first onset of cold symptoms and your use of this miracle technique will have much to do with the length of time you will find yourself suffering a cold's misery. If you use this technique at the very first sign of cold symptoms, you need not suffer longer than ten minutes from the distress which accompanies the common cold.

1. If at all possible find a location where you are not likely to be interrupted. If this cannot be arranged, place yourself in a position where you will be able to withdraw into your own consciousness for a short period of time.

2. After closing your eyes, allow yourself to relax as much as your physical position will allow. With your total consciousness follow the intake and outflow of your breath and bring it to rest in the area of your head. Allow yourself to be aware of the new relaxation flowing through your body and mind.

3. Take a deep breath through your nostrils and extend your diaphragm as you inhale. Upon completion of inhalation, relax your stomach muscles completely and allow your consciousness to follow the passage of breath through your body, again bringing it to rest in the area of your head. Repeat this process three times, and with each repetition allow yourself to be more and more aware of the total relaxation which is now present throughout your mind and body.

4. Repeat the following words to yourself mentally: "Through the wisdom of my high self and with the miraculous power of my energized mind, I command that all the immune mechanisms of my body be mobilized now and completely destroy all invading bacteria which do not contribute to my attaining and maintaining

a state of perfect health. I command that my respiratory system, sinus openings, and breathing passages be immediately healed of all inflammation and are now in a state of perfect balance and health.''

5. Take a deep breath through your nostrils and extend your diaphragm as you inhale. On completion of inhalation completely relax all stomach muscles and allow your consciousness to follow the flow of breath throughout your body, bringing it to rest finally in the area of your head. Repeat this process three times and with each inhalation allow yourself to be more and more aware of the total relaxation which now occupies your mind and body.

6. Allow your consciousness to be aware of the intake and outflow of your own breathing process without making any attempt to control it. Allow yourself to sink completely into the relaxation which is now a part of your being.

7. Open your eyes and go about your daily life.

You will find that this technique cannot fail in curing the common cold. Follow the steps carefully and make the common cold a thing you may vaguely remember but never experience in fact.

FATIGUE CAN BE A WET BLANKET

Have you ever had plans for an evening and found at the end of your day that you were too tired to carry out those plans? Have you ever been too tired to enjoy yourself at a party or other gathering? If your answer to either or both of these questions is yes, the miracle technique of energized mind which follows will be of special interest to you.

Have you ever wished you could add new vitality to a loved one who was physically or mentally fatigued? Have you ever wanted to help a wife or husband who has been completely tired out by their daily work and is visibly suffering from fatigue? If you can answer yes to either or both of these questions, the miracle technique of energized mind presented here will put you in touch with your innate ability to revitalize yourself and your loved ones through the limitless power of energized mind.

Life is a wonderful gift and in order for you to enjoy that gift fully it is necessary to have an energy level that will allow you to completely enjoy every moment you live.

If you've felt that you were "stuck" with fatigue when it struck, unless you were willing to take so-called pep pills which can endanger your health with many side-effects, you were absolutely wrong. The miracle of your own energized mind knows no limits to the amount of power it places at your disposal. It places at your disposal a source of energy that is never diminished with use and will only grow stronger the more often you call upon it. Learn now to call upon the miracle power of your energized mind and unleash its limitless force for your specific purposes wherever and whenever you wish. Whether you are at home, at work, in a department store, or riding on a bus you can use the miracle power of your energized mind to banish fatigue and completely revitalize yourself and your loved ones.

YOUR FIVE MIRACLE STEPS TO UNLIMITED ENERGY

You may use this technique for yourself or your loved ones as many times during the day as you wish. You will find, however, that with regular use of this miracle technique, fatigue becomes less and less frequent in your life and in the lives of those loved ones for whom you perform these five miracle steps.

1. If at all possible find a location where you are not likely to be interrupted. If complete privacy is not practical, put yourself in a position where you are able to close your eyes and retreat into your own consciousness for a few moments.

2. After closing your eyes allow your consciousness to be aware of the intake and outflow of your breath. Make no attempt to control your breathing process, but allow yourself to be aware of the total relaxation which is beginning to flood your mind and body. Be aware that this form of relaxation is far removed from fatigue since it places at your fingertips a limitless form of relaxed energy.

3. Take a deep breath through your nostrils, extending your diaphragm as you inhale. Upon completion of inhalation completely relax your stomach muscles and allow your consciousness to follow the flow of your breath through your body, bringing it to rest finally in the area of your head. Repeat this

process three times and with each repetition allow yourself to be more and more aware of the limitless relaxed energy which is now flooding your body and mind.

While your consciousness follows the flow of unlimited energy throughout your system, repeat the following words to yourself mentally: "As oxygen flows throughout my system the wisdom of my high self directs that each of my cells shall make the ultimate use of the oxygen it carries to them. With the unlimited power of my energized mind all my fatigue, whether physical or mental, is now banished, and a limitless form of relaxed energy has taken its rightful place in my body and mind. Whatever energy I may need is at my continuous disposal."

4. In your mind's eye see your body surrounded by, filled with, and putting forth brilliant white light. Allow yourself to be aware of the fact that this brilliant white light is symbolic of the limitless relaxed energy which is now available to you. Hold this mental image for 30 seconds.

5. Open your eyes and go about your daily life.

You will find that fatigue has completely left your mind and body, and in its place is a new and limitless relaxed form of energy which is available to you at will. With this miraculous technique you need never suffer from fatigue or lack of energy again, and as with all miraculous techniques involving the miracle of metaphysical healing, you may also use this technique to benefit your loved ones. You are a magnificent creation, a creation unequaled in the amount of energy continuously available to you through the miracle of your energized mind.

YOU NEED NEVER SPEND ANOTHER SLEEPLESS NIGHT

If you have ever been one of the millions of people who spend restless nights, unable to go to sleep, or whose sleep is so disturbed that they awaken every half hour or hour and so find it impossible to awaken refreshed in the morning, what you are about to read will be of extreme interest to you. If you have ever spent as much as one dime for medications which promise to induce sleep or to relax you so that sleep will naturally follow, you have spent your money unnecessarily. It seems strange to me that the millions of people who willingly admit that they would give just about anything for one night of sound, natural sleep try to find that natural sleep by introducing prescribed or non-prescription drugs into their bodies.

Since your body has a natural inclination to be healthy you also have a natural inclination to the enjoyment of sound, undisturbed, natural sleep. A good night's sleep is your birthright by virtue of the fact that you were born a human being. If you have sought to claim that birthright through the use of pills or liquids, you have wasted your time and energy. Whenever you wish to claim a birthright the only place to look is within yourself. That is exactly where you will find your own uncanny ability to fall asleep quickly, to stay in a sound, undisturbed sleep, and to awaken fully refreshed in the morning without the use of medications whether they be prescribed or sold over the counter. The miraculous power of your own energized mind is the force which will allow you to use this birthright at will. Through the power of your energized mind and the wisdom of your high self you will never spend another sleepless night.

Whenever anyone mentions a problem with falling asleep or staying asleep, it recalls to my own mind a gentleman by the name of Ralph J. Ralph was quick to let anyone know that he felt he was in a state of perfect health. He was just as quick to admit that the one thing in his life that was far from perfect was his sleep pattern. He often found himself so uptight at the end of a business day that when it came time to retire for the evening he was unable to fall asleep.

"I've tried everything in order to get a good night's sleep. My doctor prescribed sleeping pills for me, but they left me so groggy in the morning that I felt just as tired as when I had not slept the night before.

"Anytime I'd see an ad for something that promised to help a person sleep I'd run out and buy the product. I have a new mattress, new pillows, a record player to play soothing music for me at night, and I still toss and turn, sleeping 15 minutes here, a half hour there, while in the morning I feel as if I haven't been to bed at all.

"Just tell me what I can do to get even one good night's sleep."

I gave Ralph the same technique which is presented to you in this chapter and Ralph J., the hardened insomniac, turned into a sound and healthy sleeper. Ralph was more than willing to try the technique of metaphysical healing even if it only promised him a good night's sleep. The fact that the miracle technique of metaphysical healing through the use of energized mind was guaranteed to give him not one good night's sleep, but a good night's sleep every night was like icing on the cake as far as Ralph was concerned.

It was about 18 months ago that Ralph first used the miracle of metaphysical healing and when I spoke with him seven weeks ago, he informed me that he had not spent a sleepless night since he had first begun using the miracle technique of energized mind for the cure of insomnia and sleeplessness.

"You really ought to share this technique with everybody. I could have saved myself a lot of money that I spent on new mattresses, pillows, and all the other products that promised to give me a good night's sleep, if I had only known about the miracle of metaphysical healing earlier.

"I could have also saved myself an awful lot of money on medicine. Just out of curiosity I figured up my drug bills the other day and found that since I'm sleeping soundly every night, my drug bills have decreased by 85 percent. I guess a lot of companies that manufacture sleeping pills wouldn't be too happy if you published this miracle technique, but there would be millions of people completely overjoyed to find a safe natural way of getting a perfect night's sleep and still waking refreshed in the morning."

I wish all those drug companies well and for all of you who have ever suffered a sleepless night, the miraculous technique which will make those sleepless nights things of the past is presented for you here. Learn the technique now so that you may take advantage of your natural birthright, the right to sound, healthy, undisturbed sleep.

YOUR MIRACULOUS TECHNIQUE FOR THE CURE OF INSOMNIA AND SLEEPLESSNESS

This miraculous technique should be used just after retiring for the night. As with all the miraculous techniques of metaphysical healing presented in this book, if you wish to use this miraculous technique for a loved one, simply insert your loved one's name in the appropriate places.

1. When you have retired for the evening lie flat on your back, close your eyes, and for a moment watch your own breathing. Give your full attention to the intake and outflow of your breath but make no attempt to control this process. Allow your con-

sciousness to be totally aware of the new relaxation which is flowing into your body and mind.

2. Take a deep breath through your nostrils, and following your inhalation completely relax your stomach muscles. Repeat this process three times and with each repetition allow yourself to be more and more conscious of the total relaxation filling your mind and body.

3. Use the miracle of your mental motion picture and form an image of the muscles of your body on the screen of your mind. Repeat the following words to yourself mentally: "Through the wisdom of my high self I am aware of the total relaxation making its way through my body and mind. Through the force of energized mind I command that all the muscles of my body shall be free of all unnecessary tension and stress and will be in complete harmony within themselves and with all other systems of my body. I command that all systems of my body become relaxed and slow normally in their processes."

As you are repeating these words mentally to yourself see the muscles in the image you have projected on your mental screen become relaxed and elongated as all unnecessary tension leaves them and relaxation reigns throughout your body.

4. Take a deep breath through your nostrils and completely relax your stomach muscles. Allow your consciousness to follow the flow of this breath through your body and bring it to rest finally in the area of your head. Repeat this process three times and with each repetition feel your muscles relax even more completely as all unnecessary tension leaves your body and mind.

5. Flood your inner consciousness with the color of midnight blue. This is the color of the sky at the time of midnight. Repeat the following words to yourself mentally: "I will my consciousness into the universal blueprint of midnight blueness. As I relax into this color I feel all tension leaving my body and mind and float naturally off into sound, safe, undisturbed sleep until I wake completely refreshed in the morning."

6. Allow yourself to drift off, floating into sound, safe, natural sleep.

You now have a simple, but miraculous, five minute technique which will cure all insomnia and sleeplessness through the miracle of metaphysical healing. You need never spend another sleepless night.

DON'T WATCH YOUR LIFE GO UP IN SMOKE

One thing you will not find advertised on radio or TV any longer is cigarettes. In fact, radio and television are now involved in the effort to encourage people to stop smoking. Messages designed to encourage non-smoking can be seen on TV, ranging in form from cartoons with a serious moral all the way to messages from individuals suffering from lung cancer.

Radio and television both provide their audiences with an address where people can write if they desire tips on how to quit smoking. At the root of all techniques offered the general public for the purpose of quitting smoking is individual willpower. The technique you will learn in this chapter does not at all depend on willpower, but on the irresistible force of your own energized mind. You will stop smoking because you will achieve contact with your high self which, through the force of energized mind, will completely abolish your desire to smoke since smoking is not compatible with the natural inclination of your body to be healthy. You can quit smoking now. You can also use the miracle of metaphysical healing to help any of your loved ones stop smoking today.

Whenever I hear anyone speak about the difficulty involved in quitting smoking, Kevin L. pops into my mind. Kevin had been a heavy smoker for 15 years, inhaling on the average of three and one half packs of cigarettes per day. He was a man under considerable pressure in the business world and rationalized that smoking helped him withstand the tension that he might not be able to cope with if he did not smoke.

When Kevin began experiencing severe chest pains he quickly made an appointment with his physician. The diagnosis was angina pectoris and a physical system under severe mental stress. Kevin's doctor advised him to stop smoking immediately since it was felt that smoking would do further injury to Kevin's circulatory system and heart.

"He might as well have told me to stop breathing for my health. I know I should quit smoking, but it has become such a habit that I don't feel I really can stop.

"That doesn't seem to leave me with much of an alternative,

does it? Anyway, I didn't think I had much of an alternative before my friend told me about the miracle of metaphysical healing. I want you to teach me this miraculous technique I've been told about that will allow me to quit smoking entirely.''

Kevin and I talked about the miracle of metaphysical healing that would allow him to give up smoking not in a matter of months, weeks, or days, but in a matter of hours. The same miraculous technique of metaphysical healing which allowed Kevin to give up smoking after 15 years of three and one half packs a day is presented for your benefit in this chapter and will work just as certainly for you as it has for Kevin L. and so many others.

Don't waste another minute of your life wishing you could stop smoking. Don't waste any more time thinking about why you should quit smoking and rationalizing about why you can't quit smoking. The technique presented for you here cannot fail. It is a foolproof method of the miracle of metaphysical healing that is guaranteed to cure you of all desire to smoke.

Life is a very precious gift—don't watch yours go up in smoke. Begin now. Practice the miraculous technique given to you below, and stop smoking today.

YOUR MIRACLE TECHNIQUE FOR THE CURE OF THE DESIRE FOR AND HABIT OF SMOKING

As with all knowledge presented to you in the miraculous techniques given to you in this book, the miracle technique presented here can be used by you for your own benefit or for the benefit of any of your loved ones. If you are using this miracle technique to cure a loved one of the desire and habit of smoking, simply insert that loved one's name whenever appropriate.

Repeat this exercise five times a day at regular intervals. It is a foolproof method and cannot fail to cure you and your loved ones of the desire and habit of smoking.

1. If at all possible select a location where you are not likely to be disturbed. If privacy is not practical, position yourself so that you may close your eyes and for a moment withdraw into your own consciousness.

2. Allow your consciousness to be totally aware of the intake and outflow of your own breath, but make no attempt to control

the process. Let your consciousness be totally aware of the new relaxation beginning to flood your body and mind.

3. Take a deep breath through your nostrils, being sure to extend your diaphragm as you inhale. On completion of inhalation relax your stomach muscles completely, and follow the passage of the breath through your body with your mind's eye, allowing the breath to come to rest finally in the area of your head. Repeat this process three times and with each repetition become more and more aware of the total relaxation now flooding your mind and body.

4. Repeat the following words to yourself mentally: "Through the power of my energized mind and in the wisdom of my high self I now reject all desire to smoke. I also denounce habitual smoking and withdraw any power I may have given it over my own better judgment.

"From this point on my high self through the power of my energized mind will reject all habits and desires not in keeping with the natural inclination of my mind and body to be healthy. This process will take place even when my conscious mind is engaged in other matters."

5. Create your own mental motion picture complete with the miracle of mental sound. See yourself in situations where previously you may have smoked. See and hear someone offering you a cigarette and hear yourself respond in this manner or one similar to this, "No, thank you. I have quit smoking entirely. I decided to cooperate with my own mind and body in its natural drive to keep me healthy."

"You mean you've actually stopped smoking? That's amazing. You must have some kind of willpower! How did you do it?"

"It didn't take any willpower. I used the miracle of metaphysical healing and I no longer have any desire to smoke. Neither am I compelled to smoke through habit. I have found a miracle technique that really works and I'm a happier and healthier person because of it."

6. Take a deep breath through your nostrils, being sure to extend your diaphragm while you inhale. On completion of your inhalation completely relax your stomach muscles and allow your consciousness to follow the passage of your breath through

your body, bringing it to rest finally in the area of your head. Repeat this process three times and with each repetition allow yourself to be more and more aware of the total and complete relaxation which now floods your body and mind.

7. For a moment watch your intake and outflow of breath without making any attempt to control it. Allow yourself to become more and more aware of the total and complete relaxation which entirely fills your body and mind.

8. Open your eyes and go about your daily life.

Just as Kevin L. was able to stop smoking through the use of this miracle technique, you, too, will be able to stop smoking within a matter of hours. Through the use of this miraculous technique you will also be able to help any of your loved ones quit smoking in a few short hours instead of weeks or months.

Remember with this miraculous technique for metaphysical healing you cannot fail to lose all desire for smoking and break the chain of all habitual smoking. Stop setting fire to the gift of life. Begin today to use this miraculous technique and celebrate your body's own natural inclination to keep you in perfect health.

With these miraculous techniques now available to you in your mental medicine cabinet you will be able to use the miracle of metaphysical healing to an even greater extent in your life. You are truly a magnificent creation and with the miracle techniques for metaphysical healing presented to you here, you cannot fail to attain the natural state of perfect health which your body and mind strive for constantly.

eight

Metaphysical Healing
Brings Quick Cures
for Longstanding Illness

Do you or one of your loved ones suffer from a longstanding illness which is not fatal but has introduced much suffering and inconvenience into your daily living? The term illness is used here not only to encompass medically recognized diseases, but also includes such maladies as allergies and long-term chronic discomforts. It does not require "the eye of an eagle" to see that many phases of mass communications would have you believe that such illnesses are inherent in human nature itself and so must be endured and tolerated with the use of a mass variety of over-the-counter medications to aid you in your efforts. In an attempt to entertain you on the one hand, and sell products that will supposedly help you cope with these maladies on the other hand, radio, television, movies, and advertisements present over and over again the idea that you are prone to illness and discomfort. In an attempt to convince you of your frailty and your need for specific products to help you deal with the shortcomings of your own human nature statistics are quoted. One of these messages might run in part as follows, "Seven out of ten people suffer the discomforts of hay fever and hay fever-like allergies . . . ; . . . two out of four people suffer from a serious case of dandruff . . . ; . . . seven out of ten people suffer from nasal congestion resulting in headaches and post-nasal drip. . ." Messages like these help to make the general public sitting ducks in fertile ground for the development of the illnesses and discomforts of which they speak.

In this chapter you will learn the miraculous techniques of

metaphysical healing which will allow you to bring quick cures for longstanding illnesses. You will learn how you can stop paying money for the purchase of non-prescription drugs which claim to control your allergies, and instead heal yourself of those allergies through the miracle techniques of metaphysical healing. You will learn to bring the blessings of these miraculous techniques to all your loved ones who suffer from longstanding illnesses which disrupt their daily life and make it less enjoyable.

Since you already possess all the power necessary to cure yourself and your loved ones from any illness or disease, it is only necessary for you to learn the miraculous techniques which will put you in touch with your own power and provide you with failproof instructions for its use. This chapter makes those miraculous techniques yours today.

JOSEPH W. CURED HIMSELF OF EIGHT DIFFERENT ALLERGIES WITH METAPHYSICAL HEALING

It would seem that if one were going to suffer from allergies that two allergies would be more than enough. In fact, when you consider the fact that you have the power to cure yourself of all allergies, one allergy is too much. Joseph W. had a surplus of allergies. Joseph was an unwilling and uninformed sufferer of the effects of *eight* different allergies. If one believed the list which Joseph carried with him, he was allergic to practically everything except air. That air, of course, had to be pure or it, too, would produce some sort of allergic reaction.

Joseph sneezed and sniffled his way through our first meeting wiping his tearing eyes and explaining to me that he had suffered from allergies since he was five years of age. Anyway, that was as far back as Joseph could remember himself, "But if my parents are right, my first allergy showed up when I was three weeks old."

Joseph unwrapped the story of his childhood for me interrupted only by the intermittent use of nasal spray "for the effects of allergies that affected his nose." According to what Joseph had been told concerning his family history, his parents and their parents had all suffered from allergies and Joseph should consider himself lucky that he only had eight different allergies instead of the 16 different allergies from which his mother suffered or the 14 varieties of allergies which afflicted his father.

"As far back as I can remember our house was like a drugstore.

We had pills and liquids to combat the negative effects of anything. Believe it or not, we even had a pill to fight the bad effects of taking too many pills. That sounds like a joke, but, believe me, it's true.

"I've been the gamut as far as medical treatment for these allergies is concerned, but so far nothing has really worked. A few medications gave me some temporary relief, but I quickly grew accustomed to them and their effectiveness wore off.

"I'd like to learn the miraculous techniques for the cure of allergies which several of my friends have told me you are willing to share with people who seriously want help. You won't meet anyone more serious about being helped than I am. I'm so tired of a stuffed up head, runny eyes, and a post-nasal drip that I wish I could put in for a whole new body. I know that I can't do that but I also know that I can and am asking your help. Please teach me about metaphysical healing so I can get rid of these allergies once and for all."

Joseph had sneezed his way through half the box of tissues which he had brought with him. He never took his red and swollen eyes off me as I began to explain the miraculous techniques of metaphysical healing which would make his allergies a thing of the past. He listened intently, and when I had finished speaking he asked if he might repeat to me what he had heard in order to make sure that he understood completely the technique he was to use to benefit from the miracle of metaphysical healing. His allergies had not affected his memory one bit and when both Joseph and I were satisfied that he understood the instructions he was to follow, he left with a promise that he would contact me as soon as all eight allergies had been cured.

Five weeks later I received a phone call from Joseph.

"I just got a clean bill of health from two allergy specialists and I guess even more importantly from myself. No more allergies. I waited until all the test results were back before calling you even though I knew all the tests would be negative. You would've heard from me two weeks ago if it wasn't for the fact that I wanted the test results to make it official."

I shared Joseph's excitement. I also teased him a little about his use of nasal spray and tissues.

"What are you going to do with all the extra time that you'll have now that you don't have to use nasal sprays and so many tissues?"

"You may think you're kidding, but you know something? I really do have a lot more time. For the first time I can remember in ages I can read a book without looking through runny eyes or taking time out to spray my nose so I could breathe.

"Thanks an awful lot for teaching me about metaphysical healing. I wish there were some way you could let everyone know about this miraculous technique. Maybe someday you can write a book about it or something. Anyway, thanks an awful lot. I sure am glad I found out about the miracle of metaphysical healing."

I hear from Joseph W. every now and then and he is still enjoying an allergy-free life made possible by the miraculous techniques of metaphysical healing which he learned more than two years ago.

You can now learn the same miraculous technique of metaphysical healing which worked for Joseph W. and hundreds of other people who suffered from a variety of allergies. The steps you are to follow are listed for you, and there is no way this miraculous technique cannot work for you if you follow the failproof instructions. Don't waste another moment of your time or use one more tissue because of allergies. Begin immediately to use this miraculous technique of metaphysical healing that will bring a cure from all allergies for you and all your loved ones.

YOUR VIDEO-MEDIC TECHNIQUE FOR THE CURE OF ALLERGIES

Repeat the following miracle technique three times a day for the cure of your allergies and those of your loved ones.

1. Select a location where you are not likely to be disturbed. If possible lie down or sit in a chair whose back is high enough to support your head.

2. Close your eyes and focus your consciousness entirely on your intake and outflow of breath. Make no attempt to control your breathing process but allow your consciousness to be aware of the increased relaxation which begins to flow through your body and mind.

3. Take a deep breath through your nostrils, being sure to extend your diaphragm as you inhale. On the completion of your inhalation completely relax your stomach muscles and allow your consciousness to follow the passage of your breath through your body and bring it to rest finally in the area of your head.

Repeat this process three times and with each repetition allow yourself to be more and more aware of the increased relaxation filling your mind and body.

4. Repeat the following words to yourself mentally: "In the wisdom of my high self and through the power of my energized mind all cells in my body which are afflicted by allergies or susceptible to allergies are at this moment being restored or replaced. I am made new through the power of the creative force which flows through the use of my energized mind. This miraculous power of my energized mind will work at all times despite the fact that my conscious mind may be engaged with other matters. The wisdom of my high self shall direct me always to complete harmony and perfect health."

5. Become a video-medic producing a mental motion picture in which you see yourself completely cured of all allergies. Add the miracle of sound to your mental motion picture and hear the reactions of your loved ones congratulating you on your complete recovery from allergies.

Be sure to include a scene in which your physician will tell you that your allergies are completely cured and that you no longer suffer from allergic reactions. Hear your doctor use the following or similar words:

"The results of all your tests and my examination show that you are completely cured of your allergies. I won't pretend to understand how this has happened but I am very glad for you that it has come about. You will no longer need any medications for allergies since you no longer suffer any form of allergic reaction."

"Thank you very much, Doctor. I appreciate your thoroughness, and, believe me, I am awfully glad that I no longer have allergies."

6. Take a deep breath through your nostrils, being sure to extend your diaphragm on inhalation. On completion of inhalation completely relax your stomach muscles and allow your consciousness to follow the passage of your breath through your body, bringing it to rest finally in the area of your head. Repeat this process three times and with each repetition allow yourself to be totally aware of the complete relaxation which now occupies your body and mind.

7. For a moment allow yourself to be completely aware of your own intake and outflow of breath without making any attempt to control the process. Again be totally aware of the new and complete relaxation which now permeates your mind and body.

8. Open your eyes and go about your daily life.

You cannot fail with this technique. Your video-medic technique for the miracle of metaphysical healing will bring you and your loved ones complete freedom from all allergies. You owe it to yourself and all your loved ones who suffer from allergies to begin using this miraculous technique today.

MAN CURES HIMSELF FROM GOUT

Many young people today may never have heard of gout, but to the thousands who suffer from this painful ailment, gout is a reality which traditional medical science does not seem able to help them escape. Many who suffer from this illness turn to folk medicine and old wives' tales and go so far as soaking their feet in chlorine bleach. This process may be very good for producing clean feet and increasing the sales of chlorine bleach, but I have never heard of one case where it actually produced a cure from gout or even the suffering which attends it.

Donald E. had suffered from gout for six years and during that time had tried his share of folk remedies and followed the instructions laid out in a number of old wives' tales. He had turned to these things in desperation since conventional medicine did not seem to be able to offer him any great hope for a cure from gout or even a prolonged alleviation of the pain and discomfort which accompanies the illness. Perhaps it was also desperation which led Donald E. to follow a friend's advice and speak with me concerning the use of metaphysical healing in order to bring him to a state of perfect health and well-being.

Donald made it clear that he was willing to try anything and I made it just as clear that the only thing I had to offer him was a means of contacting the power within himself and the techniques for using that power. I was quick to add that this was a combination that could in no way fail in giving Donald a complete cure from the gout from which he suffered.

"Just tell me what I'm supposed to do and I'll start doing it today. You can't possibly imagine how much I want to be rid of this and how badly I want to be able to walk without crutches."

I talked and Donald listened. Donald talked and I listened. At the end of our meeting we both understood what the other was saying and Donald left in an extremely optimistic state of mind.

Three weeks later a phone call came from Donald. His voice was crackling with excitement as it bubbled forth from my end of our telephone connection.

"Would you like to buy a pair of used crutches? Guess what? No more gout. My doctor says that I am completely cured not only of the gout but also of a mild kidney disease which he had suspected to be the cause of it.

"I would have called you sooner but I figured you'd want to know what the doctor had to say before you heard from me. Well, it's official, no more gout.

"That metaphysical healing is really powerful stuff. I only wish I had met you six years ago."

I didn't bother to tell Donald E. that six years prior to the time he was speaking with me I was probably in worse shape than he was with his gout. Thanks to the miracle of metaphysical healing he or no one else could suspect that fact without being told.

You are now in a position to bring the miracle of metaphysical healing to any of your loved ones who suffer from gout. It goes without saying, of course, that if you happen to be one of the thousands of gout sufferers then you can also use the following miracle technique for yourself. Join Donald and the hundreds of others like him who have been cured from gout with the use of the miraculous technique presented here.

YOUR ENERGIZED MIND TECHNIQUE FOR THE CURE OF GOUT

Repeat the following miracle technique three times a day. It is a failproof method to bring the miracle of metaphysical healing to you and all your loved ones who suffer from gout.

1. Select a location where you are not likely to be interrupted. Lie down or sit in a chair with a back high enough to support your head.

2. Close your eyes and for a moment focus your consciousness

completely on your intake and outflow of breath without making any attempt to control it. Allow yourself to be aware of the relaxation which is beginning to fill your mind and body.

3. Take a deep breath through your nostrils and be sure to extend your diaphragm as you inhale. Upon completion of inhalation completely relax your stomach muscles and allow your consciousness to follow the breath through your body and bring it to rest finally in the area of your head. Repeat this process three times and with each repetition allow yourself to become more and more aware of the increased relaxation now filling your body and mind.

4. Repeat the following words to yourself mentally: "In the wisdom of my high self and through the power of my energized mind I command that all cells in my body afflicted with the illness of gout will now be restored or replaced. I command also that all cells in my body suffering from any disease which may have brought about the condition of gout also be restored or replaced immediately. Through the power of energized mind my high self shall continuously direct the miracle of metaphysical healing on my behalf even though my conscious mind may be engaged with other matters."

5. Produce your own mental motion picture and add the miracle of sound to your production. See yourself walking without aid and completely free of all pain and symptoms of gout.

See and hear yourself conversing with your loved ones sharing each other's enthusiasm at the fact that you have been cured completely of gout.

See and hear yourself in your physician's office as your physician speaks the following or similar words: "My examination and all test results show that you no longer suffer from gout or any of the diseases which brought it about. You will now be able to discontinue all medication."

"Thank you, doctor. I'm very glad myself that I no longer have gout or any disease that would cause it."

6. Take a deep breath through your nostrils, being sure to extend your diaphragm as you inhale. Upon completion of inhalation, completely relax your stomach muscles and allow your consciousness to follow your breath through your body and bring it to rest finally in the area of your head. Repeat this proc-

ess three times and with each repetition allow yourself to become more and more aware of the total relaxation which is now flooding both your mind and body.

7. For a moment focus your consciousness on your own intake and outflow of breath but make no attempt to control this process. Allow yourself to become more and more aware of the total relaxation which completely fills your body and mind.

8. Open your eyes and go about your daily life.

If you or any of your loved ones has suffered from gout you have already suffered long enough. Begin today to use this miracle technique of energized mind in order to bring the miracle of metaphysical healing to yourself and your loved ones so that you may all share the blessing of perfect health which is your birthright.

MILLIONS OF WOMEN SUFFER UNNECESSARY PAIN EACH MONTH

Each month millions of women suffer the pain and discomfort of menstrual cramps. Thousands of these women purchase non-prescription medications which promise to relieve the pain of menstrual cramps and plan to take this medication each month for this purpose. The greatest majority of these women, $99^9/_{10}$ percent, would be happy if the pain associated with menstrual cramps could be alleviated each month and give little or no thought to obtaining a cure for the cause of the pain they suffer. The majority of women have come to accept monthly menstrual cramps as an unfortunate but necessary component of womanhood.

If you are one of the women who suffer from menstrual cramps each month, or if any of your loved ones can be counted in this number, the time for you to learn that this is unnecessary suffering is long overdue. You and your loved ones need never suffer again from monthly menstrual cramps. Through the miracle of metaphysical healing you can make menstrual cramps a thing of the past. To accomplish this feat it will not be necessary for you to spend another cent, you need only follow the miraculous exercise of energized mind that is presented for you later in this chapter. If you follow the step by step failproof method you can rest assured that you have already suffered your last bout with menstrual cramps.

SEVERE MENSTRUAL CRAMPS COST A WOMAN HER JOB

Eilene R. came to visit me three days after she was fired from her job. She had been employed only four months when her supervisor decided he could no longer contend with Eilene's absenteeism. Since Eilene had been employed as a nurse's aid and her absence meant that the particular shift for which she was scheduled to work would go shorthanded at the patients' expense, Eilene was not considered a good employee in a hospital setting.

"I understand their problem and why my supervisor fired me, but it doesn't make it any easier for me to accept. I really loved that job and had been giving a lot of thought about going to nursing school. If I can't do something about these severe cramps each month, it doesn't seem likely that I could hold any job."

Eilene had run the gamut of non-prescription medications for menstrual cramps and had also taken several prescription medications in an attempt to find something that would control her pain. It seemed that finding a pain reliever only presented her with a new problem. If the pain reliever was strong enough to kill the pain Eilene experienced, it was also strong enough to affect her awareness and effectiveness as an employee. Either way Eilene had a genuine problem concerning employment.

"When I was in high school and had to be absent I could work twice as hard to make up for the work I'd missed. I'm afraid it doesn't work like that in the business world.

"I want you to teach me the metaphysical healing technique for curing my cramps once and for all. My friend, Norma N., told me that she hasn't had cramps once since she began using the miracle technique you taught her. I just wish she had told me about it before I lost my job."

We discussed the steps Eilene was to follow and she left with the statement, "It's too bad that we have to wait almost a month to find out the results. I'll let you know as soon as I know."

"Eilene, I can guarantee that this technique works. The only reason we'll have to wait a month is so you'll know that, too."

One month passed and I heard nothing from Eilene R. At the end of two and a half months I received a phone call from her.

"I'm sorry I didn't call you sooner but I wanted to make sure that I was really cured. When I didn't have any cramps two months ago I thought maybe I had just psyched myself out but last month the same thing happened, no cramps.

"I have my job back again at the hospital and I haven't missed a day in six weeks. My supervisor was amazed when I told her what had happened and then she decided that the medical world is still learning.

"Thank you very much for teaching me that miraculous technique."

I ran into Eilene R. about eight months after her phone call. She was still employed on her job, had received two promotions, had not experienced menstrual cramps since she used the miracle of metaphysical healing to cure herself of their cause.

YOUR MIRACULOUS TECHNIQUE OF ENERGIZED MIND FOR THE CURE OF MENSTRUAL CRAMPS

If you are one of the many women who still suffer from menstrual cramps, or if one of your loved ones is included in that number, this exercise will be of extreme benefit to you. Repeat this exercise three times a day for yourself, for your loved ones, or for both of you.

As with all metaphysical healing techniques presented to you in this book, if you are performing this exercise for both yourself and a loved one or loved ones simply include yourself and the name or names of your loved ones each time you perform the specific miracle technique. It is not necessary to perform this miraculous technique or any other miracle technique in this book separately for each individual for whom you intend the benefit of the miracle of metaphysical healing. As you perform the prescribed miracle exercises you may include yourself and as many of your loved ones as you wish.

1. Select a location where you are not likely to be interrupted. Lie down or sit in a chair whose back is high enough to support your head.

2. Close your eyes and for a moment give your full attention to the intake and outflow of your breath without any attempt to control it. Allow your consciousness to be totally aware of the new relaxation which is beginning to flow into your mind and body.

3. Take a deep breath through your nostrils, being sure to extend your diaphragm as you inhale. Upon completion of inhalation completely relax your stomach muscles and allow your consciousness to follow your breath through your body and come to rest finally in the area of your head. Repeat this exercise three times and with each repetition become more and more aware of the total relaxation now filling your mind and body.

4. Repeat the following words to yourself mentally: "In the wisdom of my high self and through the power of my energized mind all cells in my body which are experiencing or subject to menstrual cramps are now being restored or replaced. I further command that any of my cells diseased or damaged which may contribute to menstrual cramps are also being restored or replaced this very moment. In union with the very principle to which my body and mind direct themselves I command that I am now perfectly healthy and that all organs and systems of my body are working in harmony within themselves and are harmonious with all other systems of my body.

"The power of my energized mind in the wisdom of my high self is constantly directing the miracle of metaphysical healing to my body and mind even when my conscious mind may be occupied with other matters."

5. Produce a mental motion picture and see yourself speaking with your loved ones telling them how happy you are that you no longer suffer from menstrual cramps. Add the miracle of sound and repeat the following words or words with the same meaning.

"It's really great not to suffer from menstrual cramps any longer. Would you believe I have not had cramps since I started using the technique for the miracle of metaphysical healing? It really works."

6. Take a deep breath through your nostrils, being sure to extend your diaphragm as you inhale. On completion of your inhalation allow your consciousness to follow the breath through your body and bring it to rest finally in the area of your head. Let your consciousness be totally aware of the complete relaxation which now fills your body and mind.

7. For a moment allow yourself to be totally aware of the intake and outflow of your breath with no attempt to control it. Again

be completely and totally aware of the fact that complete relaxation now permeates your body and mind.

8. Open your eyes and go about your daily life.

With the knowledge of metaphysical healing provided for you in this exercise and the limitless power which is yours by virtue of the fact that you are a human being, you will never know the pain or discomfort of menstrual cramps again. You may bring the same blessing of metaphysical healing to all your loved ones who suffer the pain and discomfort of menstrual cramps simply by including them also as you perform this miraculous technique. Do not allow your loved ones or yourself to spend another unnecessary moment in discomfort or pain. Begin to use this miraculous technique today.

CURING ILLNESS IS ONE THING, PREVENTING IT IS ANOTHER

We are all magnificent creations. The fact that our creator has endowed us with the ability to restore ourselves to perfect health no matter what the disease or illness we suffer is a truth which fills me with a sense of wonder and a constant desire to celebrate the gift of life. When I consider further that that same creator also placed in human beings the unlimited ability to preserve their perfect health and prevent illness, disease, and injury, I stand in sheer awe of the magnificent and limitless power given to the human race.

It is only natural that we should be expected to do everything within our limitless power to preserve the harmony of perfect health within us once we have attained that gift. Any gift which is valued is taken care of and kept from harm's way. The gift of perfect health is no exception. It is the concern of each individual human being to use the miraculous and unlimited power present in humanness itself in order to prevent disease, illness, and injury from doing damage to the most precious of all gifts, the gift of life.

Since you already possess the unlimited power capable of preventing all disease, illness, and injury it is only necessary for you to learn the methods of tapping this power and the means of putting it to its greatest use. The miraculous exercise for preventive metaphysical healing which follows will allow you to do exactly that. Follow the failproof steps in the miraculous exercise given to you here and you will find that disease, illness, injury become only faint memories in your past.

YOUR ENERGIZED MIND TECHNIQUE FOR PREVENTIVE METAPHYSICAL HEALING

This miraculous technique is guaranteed to protect the health which you now enjoy and to maintain the gift of perfect health once you have attained it. It adds strength and vitality to healthy cells, making it impossible for disease or illness to affect them. Once you have achieved the state of perfect health through the use of the miracle of metaphysical healing, the miraculous technique will allow you to preserve your perfect state of health through the use of preventive metaphysical healing.

Repeat this miraculous exercise three times a day for yourself and your loved ones and you will find that illness, disease, and injury become alien to you and them.

1. Select a location in which you are not likely to be interrupted. Lie down or sit in a chair whose back is high enough to support your head.

2. Close your eyes and give your full attention to the intake and outflow of your breath with no attempt to control the process. Allow your consciousness to be totally aware of the new relaxation beginning to fill your mind and body.

3. Take a deep breath through your nostrils, being sure to extend your diaphragm as you inhale. Upon completion of inhalation allow your consciousness to follow the breath through your body and bring it to rest finally in the area of your head. Repeat this process three times and with each repetition allow yourself to be more and more aware of the total relaxation now filling your mind and body.

4. Repeat the following words to yourself mentally: "In the wisdom of my high self and through the force of my energized mind I stand in full consciousness and appreciation for the gift of health which I enjoy. In the total awareness of the fact that I have only that which I appreciate I say my thank you for the gift of health by living my life fully. Backed by the power of my energized mind I will that my life be constantly in accord with

the maintenance of complete harmony in a perfect state of physical and mental health which I will to enjoy."

5. Take a deep breath through your nostrils, being sure to extend your diaphragm as you inhale. Upon completion of your inhalation allow your consciousness to follow the path of your breath and bring it to rest finally in the area of your head. Repeat this process three times, allowing your consciousness to be totally and completely aware of the complete relaxation which now fills your body and mind.

6. For a moment place your total attention on the intake and outflow of your breath with no attempt to control the process. Again be completely aware that perfect relaxation now fills your body and mind.

7. Open your eyes and go about your daily life.

Preventive medicine has become an accepted discipline within the realms of traditional medicine. The miracle of preventive metaphysical healing is an extremely valuable area in the field of metaphysical healing itself.

You now have everything necessary to keep yourself in a state of perfect health and your life in complete harmony with that state of perfect health. Begin to use this miracle technique today in order that you and your loved ones may show appreciation for the gift of health by giving that gift total protection.

This chapter has put at your disposal the means by which you can bring quick cures to all longstanding illnesses for yourself and your loved ones. It has also given you the knowledge necessary to protect and maintain the precious gift of perfect health once you have achieved it. Begin today to use this miraculous information for your benefit and the benefit of those you love.

nine

Your Miracle Power
of Metaphysical Healing
in Emergency Situations

Have you ever been involved in an emergency situation which centered around sickness or injury? Have you ever been notified that one of your loved ones had been taken to a hospital following an accident or acute onset of illness? If your answer to either or both of these questions is no, chances are that at some point in your future you will be called upon to respond in an emergency situation involving someone's health. Will you know what to do when that situation arises?

If your answer to either or both of the two questions is yes, then you already know that a feeling of helplessness in an emergency situation is an extremely frustrating experience. If you did everything you could according to the rules of first aid and traditional medicine and still wished that there was more you could have done, you most likely still experience the gnawing frustration of a feeling of inadequacy. With the miracle techniques of metaphysical healing which you will learn in this chapter you will never be or feel helpless again in case of emergencies. You will have the miracle methods at your disposal that will allow you to prevent serious aftereffects of injuries and illnesses which have an acute onset.

From the time we were children the majority of us have been exposed to the term first aid. You, just as I was, were probably encouraged to take a first aid course and perhaps even extend your knowledge with an advanced course at some future time. It would be foolish to deny the benefit of first aid treatment in emergency cases since what happens immediately following the acute onset of illness or an accident may seriously affect the final outcome of the patient's condition. I personally believe that everyone should have a knowledge of first aid since in many cases of accidents and acute onset of illness, a person with appropriate first aid training may prevent complications following either of these incidents and may in some circumstances even prevent the victim's death. The National Red Cross and many schools and organizations offer first aid courses to the general public and every individual can benefit from the knowledge gained by successful completion of such a course.

You are now in a position to learn a new kind of first aid treatment which will work hand-in-hand with the knowledge you will gain in an ordinary first aid class. This new first aid consists of several miraculous techniques for the use of the miracle of metaphysical healing in emergency situations. If you are present when accident or illness strike, you may use the emergency techniques of metaphysical healing as a complement to ordinary first aid treatment. Just as important, and in some cases more important, you may also use the miracle techniques of metaphysical healing for emergency situations in which you are not present. The unlimited power unleashed by these miracle techniques knows no boundary in time or space and you can aid a victim separated from you by even thousands of miles. With the use of the miracle of metaphysical healing you can prevent serious aftereffects of accidents and illnesses, such as heart attacks, which have a very quick onset. The miraculous techniques you will learn in this chapter will enable you to stand not as a helpless bystander but as a ready and powerful aid to help yourself and your loved ones in all emergencies involving accident and illness.

WOMAN USES METAPHYSICAL HEALING TO PREVENT SERIOUS BURNS

Many of the accidents which occur in a normal day involve burns sustained by people at work, at home, or at play. Accidents involving burns are severely painful to the victim and more often than not leave serious aftereffects. With the miracle of metaphysical healing you can alleviate the pain, prevent serious aftereffects, and promote healing in all burn cases involving yourself or a loved one. In order to make use of this ability it will be necessary for you to learn the miraculous techniques presented to you in this chapter by heart as soon as possible. In order to make use of the miracle of metaphysical healing in emergency cases it is necessary that the miraculous techniques which will direct your unlimited power of energized mind be available to you instantly at all times.

Jean B. attended a class I taught involving the use of metaphysical healing in emergency cases. In class Jean gave her undivided attention and made it evident that she had studied diligently in order that she might master the miraculous techniques of energized mind that would allow her to be of unlimited value to herself and her loved ones in any crisis involving accident or illness.

Eight months after Jean had completed the course she paid me a visit.

"I know you must be surprised to see me but I just had to come by and tell you about my niece."

Jean B. went on to say that three months ago her four year old niece had suffered first and some second degree burns on her shoulders, chest and stomach. The burns were the result of a four year old's curiosity concerning lobsters. Brenda had been watching her mother and aunts preparing a dinner where lobster was to be the main course for a family reunion.

Several large pots containing boiling water and a number of lobsters each were present on the stove and the kitchen was crowded with the family's women who were talking and carrying out their individual assignments for the preparation of what should have been an extremely happy occasion. No one knew exactly how it happened but conversation was brought to a halt by a child's scream and the sound of water and several hard objects striking the floor. Brenda, age four, had climbed on a chair and pulled a pot of boiling water down on her in an attempt to see the lobsters in the pots. What followed would easily have passed for complete chaos.

Brenda was crying in long breath-gasping sobs, her mother appeared to be in shock, crying and laughing hysterically at the same time, as one of Brenda's aunts picked her up and shouted for someone to turn the cold water on in the kitchen sink. Jean searched for the cold water tap, turned the water on, and began to recite out loud the metaphysical healing exercise for the miraculous healing of burns.

"Get me a blanket," shouted Brenda's aunt who was holding her body under the cold running water in the kitchen sink.

"Jean, pull your car up around front of the house and blow your horn when you're ready. We have to get her to the hospital right away. I'll hold her under this cold water until I hear the horn.''

The horn blew and Brenda's aunt wrapped Brenda in a blanket and ran with her to the car. Twenty-five minutes later they were at the hospital's emergency room and Brenda was in the hands of a physician.

''It was only 40 minutes before the doctor who was treating Brenda came out of the emergency room, but it seemed like two hours. He said that Brenda was going to be okay and then asked what had happened. As I told him the story he stared at me, his mouth half open in disbelief.''

''The child is not burned badly enough to have had a pot of boiling water spilled across the front of her body. Was she wearing additional clothes when it happened?''

''I explained that she had not been wearing any additional clothes when the accident occurred. I also expressed my relief that she was going to be all right.''

The doctor returned to the subject of Brenda's clothes when the accident occurred. ''The child has suffered mainly first degree burns with a very small area showing one second degree burn. If what you say happened did happen, it would be reasonable to expect large areas of second degree burns and some places where the burns were almost third degree in severity.''

Jean went on to tell me about the doctor's amazement at the fact that Brenda had not been burned more severely and then started to talk about metaphysical healing.

''The metaphysical healing techniques which I learned from you prevented Brenda from being more seriously injured than she was. She has one slight scar about the size of a dime in spite of the fact that according to the doctor she should have been burned badly enough to have still been in the hospital.''

I learned that Brenda's stay in the hospital had lasted only three days and that those three days were more for observation than for treatment. Brenda was fine and the dime-sized scar on her left shoulder was hardly noticeable. The miracle of metaphysical healing had prevented an accident from turning into a tragedy.

''I guess I should have come to see you and tell you about this sooner, but I left for California two days after Brenda was released from the hospital.

"I could never put into words the value of the techniques of metaphysical healing. If I never have occasion to use what I learned again my time and effort have been well-spent. Thank you for me and thank you for Brenda."

The miracle technique of energized mind which Jean used with Brenda in this time of crisis is presented for you here. I sincerely hope, just as I know you do, that you will never have an occasion arise where it is necessary to use this miracle technique. I realize, however, that it is much wiser to be prepared in case of a crisis instead of wishing after the crisis has passed that you had been prepared. For yourself and all those whom you love these miraculous techniques are a guaranteed form of insurance that no accident or injury will leave serious aftereffects to mar your life or the lives of any of your loved ones.

Learn this technique today for yourself and all those you love. Learn it for the simple reason that you love them.

YOUR ULTRA-MIND TECHNIQUE TO COOL AND CURE BURNS

The miraculous technique which follows is guaranteed to take the heat out of burns and leave the burn victim free of serious aftereffects. It is designed for use in emergency situations and can also be used in situations where, due to circumstances, metaphysical healing of a burn victim was not started immediately. In cases where the miracle of metaphysical healing has been delayed you may wish to use this technique as often as three times a day.

1. Repeat the following words either aloud or to yourself mentally: "In the wisdom of my high self and with the cooling power of my ultra-mind I command that the cells of my body now repel all damage due to burns. I command that the cells newly-created in me be directed to restore and replace any cell of my body in the least bit affected by a burn.

"In accord with its natural inclination to attain a state of perfect health, my body will throw off through the force of ultra-mind any circumstance or illness which impedes this goal."

2. Take a deep breath through your nostrils, extending your diaphragm as you inhale. Upon completion of inhalation, relax

your stomach muscles completely and allow yourself to be aware of the new relaxation and ultimate power flowing through your body and mind. Repeat this process three times. Consult your physician immediately in order to document the miracle of metaphysical healing and receive any additional aid conventional medicine can offer you.

Commit this technique to memory and learn it by heart so that in case of an emergency it will fill your mind as naturally as breath fills your body. As Jean B. so aptly phrased her own feelings concerning this method, know that if you use it only once in your lifetime your time and effort in committing it to memory and learning these miraculous steps by heart will be well worth the energy you expend to do so.

BROKEN BONES AND METAPHYSICAL HEALING

One of the most common injuries in childhood is that of bone fractures. Broken arms and legs present emergency situations pretty regularly in the lives of parents, teachers, and all those who deal with young children.

In addition to being extremely painful, a broken bone, aided by conventional medicine, still takes weeks and even months to heal completely. With the miracle technique of energized mind which you will learn in this chapter you can accelerate the healing process 25 or even 50 times its normal rate. This miraculous technique will also provide freedom from pain even while the bone remains unset. When the bone has been properly set by a physician the miracle of metaphysical healing will immediately start the accelerated healing process into action and the knitting of the fracture will take place at an astounding rate.

Another area of our population often presented with the emergency of broken bones is our senior citizens. It is an extremely well-accepted fact that the knitting of bones in fractures involving the elderly is extremely time-consuming. The same miracle technique which will allow you to work in an emergency situation in dealing with fractures involving children will also equip you to deal with the broken bones of senior citizens. The miracle power of metaphysical healing does not discriminate according to age groups and its power works just as effectively for the very young or the very old.

Of course you are aware that emergencies often arise where people of all ages may suffer from fractures. By using the miraculous technique of metaphysical healing you will be able to stop pain and greatly accelerate healing in all cases involving fractures. Whether that fracture involves one of the small bones in the hand known as metacarpals or the large bone in the thigh known as the femur, the miracle of metaphysical healing will bring painless, speedy, and miraculous recovery to all who suffer the agony of broken bones.

YOUR MIRACLE TECHNIQUE OF ENERGIZED MIND FOR THE HEALING OF FRACTURES

You may use this miraculous technique for yourself or any of your loved ones. If you are present when an emergency arises involving a broken bone use this technique immediately. If you learn of the injury sometime after it has occurred, use this technique three times a day.

1. Repeat the following words aloud or to yourself mentally: "In the full awareness of my high self and through the power of my energized mind I direct that my unlimited energies for metaphysical healing be directed to the complete alleviation of pain associated with this injury and to greatly increase the healing energies of this broken bone. I command that this bone shall be restored to a state of perfect health, leaving no after-effects as a result of this fracture."

2. Take a deep breath through the nostrils, extending the diaphragm as you inhale. Upon completion of inhalation relax your stomach muscles completely and allow your consciousness to follow the breath through your body, bringing it to rest in the area of your head. Repeat this process three times, allowing yourself to be totally aware of the unlimited energy being released for the alleviation of pain associated with this injury and the accelerated healing process of this bone fracture.

When you use this miraculous technique you will find very quickly that it provides a foolproof method through metaphysical healing to break the time barrier of normal bone knitting and bring about a speedy and complete healing of any fracture for which its miraculous power is used.

HEART ATTACKS CREATE EMERGENCY SITUATIONS

Every reader of this book will find the metaphysical healing technique which follows of extreme personal interest and benefit. For the hundreds of thousands of people who have been present when a loved one has suffered a heart attack the miraculous technique presented here can offer the reader a secure knowledge that he or she will now be able to play an active role in the recovery of the heart attack victim. The reader who learns this failproof method of ultra-mind need never be paralyzed into inactivity by fear when a heart attack creates an emergency situation. Whether you use the miraculous technique of ultra-mind for yourself or for a loved one it will restore perfect health and harmony to the heart and circulatory system.

WOMAN USES ULTRA-MIND TO RESTORE A HEART ATTACK VICTIM

Phyllis C. had enrolled in my classes as a result of her husband's family history of heart ailment and heart attack. It was not unusual for Phyllis to remain after class to ask additional questions and to reassure herself that she understood completely the metaphysical healing techniques which had been discussed during the class period.

Phyllis had spoken many times in the presence of the class concerning her terrible feelings of inadequacy which she experienced when her husband suffered his first heart attack in her presence.

"I could never put into words the way I felt when he grabbed for his chest and fell unconscious on the floor. I thank God that I had the presence of mind to call an ambulance, but it seemed that there should have been something I could have done while waiting for the ambulance to arrive. I felt as if he might die right in front of me and I was powerless to do anything to prevent it."

It was obvious that Phyllis C. really applied herself to her studies and put an extra emphasis on the techniques of ultra-mind for the miraculous treatment of heart attacks. At the completion of the course Phyllis stated that she sincerely hoped she would never have to use the miracle technique she had learned, but she felt confident that if she was placed in an emergency situation those miraculous techniques of metaphysical healing would allow her to help the stricken victim.

Seven months after Phyllis had completed her course she paid me a visit. Phyllis wasted no time in telling me that her husband had suffered another heart attack, an unfortunate fact in itself, and to add to the unfortunate circumstances of that heart attack, James C. had been stricken at work and taken to a hospital. Two hours had passed before Phyllis was able to be contacted concerning her husband's condition.

"I was scared, but I wasn't half as scared as I would have been had I not known about the ultra-mind technique for the treatment of heart attacks. It bothered me at first that so much time had elapsed since the heart attack had struck, but I remembered what I had learned in class and decided to make time count now. I began immediately to use the miraculous techniques of ultra-mind to bring healing and perfect health to James' heart.

"I also started working immediately using this technique to prevent aftereffects as a result of his heart attack."

The complete facts of this case were unfolded to me as Phyllis and I talked. At first doctors felt that James had suffered a rather severe heart attack and had placed him in an intensive care unit. Doctors had given him a less than 50-50 chance of pulling through.

Three hours after James had been placed in the intensive care unit he regained consciousness and appeared to be making steady strides on a march back to health. When his doctor stopped in to see him an hour later it was decided that James could be taken out of the oxygen tent and moved from the intensive care unit.

"The doctor didn't really say much, but anyone could see by the look on his face that he was really surprised to find James that much improved. One of the nurses told me it was most unusual for any heart attack victim to leave the intensive care unit that quickly."

Phyllis C. continued to use the miracle of ultra-mind and her husband James continued to grow in strength on a road which led to perfect health. The original prognosis of a less than 50-50 chance of James' attaining a recovery was changed when he was removed from the intensive care unit. Doctors now told Phyllis that her husband would be hospitalized approximately eight weeks and that it might be as long as four months before James could return to work. Phyllis listened and continued to perform the technique of ultra-mind which she was convinced would restore James to perfect health.

One week later doctors had another revised prognosis concerning James C. It was now felt that James might very well leave the hospital in as few as four weeks. Phyllis received the news with a light heart and again continued to use the miraculous techniques of ultra-mind as an additional tool in James C.'s recovery.

Another week went by filled with more physical examinations and special tests for James C. At the end of his second week in the hospital doctors announced to him and to his wife that he would be able to leave the hospital in one more week. It was a much amazed physician struggling to keep his professional tone of voice who told Phyllis and her husband, "In my 15 years of practice in cardiology I have never seen anyone recover from a massive heart attack so quickly. You're very lucky that your will to live is so strong and that your body has an exceptional ability for extremely rapid regeneration and recovery.

"In view of this episode I do not understand why it took you so long to recover from your first heart attack."

James left the hospital in a week and at the end of another week he was back at work on a part-time basis. That part-time basis didn't last long since James was working full-time again when only one week had elapsed.

Phyllis C. was delighted, and her husband, James, was in excellent condition. A recent physical by his physician had shown that there was no heart damage due to his second heart attack and what seemed to many of his physicians a strange fact, much of the damage done by his first heart attack had also disappeared. By his doctor's own admission James was stronger than ever.

"It's just wonderful to see him so healthy and happy again. Before he worried just as much as I did, although he didn't let it be known, that he would suffer another heart attack and that the second one would be worse than the first.

"Well, that second heart attack was worse than the first, but one thing he didn't count on and I guess I didn't count on at that time, either, was the fact that we had the miracle of metaphysical healing to help us through that emergency. I've explained the miracle technique to James and he uses it for himself now three times a day.

"Thank you for sharing the technique with me. It has meant more to my husband and me than I could ever put into words."

The same miraculous technique which worked for Phyllis C. is presented for your use in this chapter. You have only to commit this miraculous technique to memory and you will be fully prepared to handle any emergency involving heart attacks. The same technique of ultra-mind will also allow you to restore damage done by previous heart attacks and to return the heart attack victims to perfect health.

Both miraculous results will be yours through the use of the one miracle technique for metaphysical healing presented below. Learn that technique today and feel confident that you will be able to handle any emergency situation which strikes a blow to the heart and adds a heavy weight to the emotions.

YOUR ULTRA-MIND TECHNIQUE FOR THE TREATMENT OF HEART ATTACKS AND THE RESTORATION OF PERFECT HEALTH TO ALL CELLS DAMAGED BY THOSE ATTACKS

If you are using this technique during the actual time this emergency is occurring, you need only carry out steps four and five. If an hour or more has passed since the time the emergency was created it will be necessary for you to carry out the entire exercise presented here, to repeat this exercise three times a day.

1. Choose a place where you are not likely to be interrupted. Lie down or sit in a chair whose back is high enough to support your head.

2. Close your eyes and for a moment watch the intake and outflow of your own breath without making any attempt to control it. Allow yourself to be aware of the new relaxation beginning to flood your mind and body.

3. Take a deep breath through your nostrils, extending your diaphragm as you inhale. Upon completion of inhalation completely relax your stomach muscles and allow your consciousness to follow the breath throughout your body, bringing it to rest finally in the area of your head. Repeat this process three times and with each repetition allow yourself to be more and more aware of the total relaxation now flooding your mind and body.

4. Repeat the following words to yourself mentally: "In the wisdom of my high self and through the power of my ultra-mind I command that no further damage be done to the cells of my body. I further will that all cells in any way damaged or impaired due to heart ailment or heart attack will be restored or replaced through the power of my ultra-mind immediately.

"This miraculous process of metaphysical healing will take place continuously even though my conscious mind may be engaged in other matters or may fall into unconsciousness."

5. Take a deep breath through your nostrils, extending your diaphragm as you inhale. Upon completion of inhalation completely relax your stomach muscles and allow your consciousness to follow the breath throughout your body, bringing it to rest finally in the area of your head. Repeat this process three times and with each repetition allow your consciousness to be more and more aware of the total relaxation now flooding your body and mind.

Repeat the following words to yourself mentally: "Through the miraculous power of ultra-mind now filling my body and mind completely I command that I be returned to perfect health completely free of sickness, pain, and affliction."

6. For a brief moment watch your intake and outflow of breath without any attempt to control it. Again allow yourself to be aware completely of the relaxation now present throughout your body and mind.

7. Open your eyes and go about your daily life.

This miraculous technique of ultra-mind for metaphysical healing for heart attacks and all damage to the heart and circulatory system is a fail-proof method of restoring you and your loved ones to perfect health. There is no way you can fail with the use of this miraculous technique.

If you are present during the time of the emergency and use steps four and five for immediate emergency care, you may still wish to repeat the entire technique three times a day for three days as a special precaution. This is not at all unusual since in conventional medicine doctors often give prescriptions where the dosage not only allows for a cure but, moreover, kills all existing bacteria.

You may also use the miracle of metaphysical healing to prevent heart attack and heart disease. These steps are outlined for you in Chapter eight. By following them faithfully you will be able to maintain the heart and circulatory system in perfect health and safe from the assault of all disease and affliction.

You need never be helpless in any emergency situation again. The information you have gained in this chapter will allow you to be a vital and helpful force for the recovery of any individual stricken by disease or injury with such suddenness that an emergency is created. Commit these techniques to memory—they cannot fail you, and through their use you cannot fail yourself or your loved ones.

ten

How to Cure
Negative Thinking
Through Metaphysical Healing

No individual who is a habitual negative thinker can live a healthy, happy life until the disease of negative thinking has been cured. The fact may surprise you, but negative thinking is just as real a disease as cancer, arthritis, or ulcers. Your health can be torn apart by negative thoughts and the disease of negative thinking can spread to tear your entire life into pieces. Negative thinking is a disease that can kill every chance an individual has to lead a happy life without his realizing that a vicious and fatal disease is killing everything around him.

It may truly be said that every person experiences a negative thought once in a while. In this chapter you will learn how to deal with that occasional negative thought so that it will never become the horrible and fatal disease of habitual negative thinking. Your response to a negative thought will have a great deal of effect in determining whether negative thinking destroys you and your loved ones or is cast out by you as a recognized danger to your health and happiness.

Consider this fact: everything in this world once started with a thought. Thought is such a powerful form of energy that nothing can come into existence or go out of existence without its process. Your thoughts are truly the stuff your life is made of, and if those thoughts are negative you can expect a life filled with negativity. In this chapter the person who has been so unfortunate as to fill his or her life with negativity will learn the process of metaphysical healing which will cure the fatal disease of negative thinking and change the individual's entire life style. So, whether you want to learn how to prevent occasional negative thoughts from becoming habitual negative thinking, or how to cure the vicious and fatal disease of habitual negative thinking, you will find exactly what you need in this chapter. You need only follow the step-by-step exercises which will bring the miracle of metaphysical healing into your life in order to discover for yourself that you are a natural-born winner.

MAN USES THE MIRACLE OF METAPHYSICAL HEALING TO BREAK THE LOSER CYCLE

Have you ever known a man or a woman who, no matter what he or she did, seemed always to come out on the short end of the stick? This is the individual who could have everything planned to the nth degree with not even a hint that anything could go wrong and then, at the last minute, have the world turn upside down spilling plans and dreams into one chaotic mess. How this individual rects to this stressful situation will determine the ultimate outcome for that individual. If this person sits around feeling sorry for himself, wondering how in the world all this tragedy could happen to him, he will very quickly find himself in what is known as the loser cycle. Since thoughts attract like magnets, but, unlike magnets, attract like things unto themselves, this person will be pulling all kinds of negative circumstances into his life.

If, on the other hand, this individual faced with chaotic situations maintains a hopeful attitude and a sound belief that all will turn out well, he will find that he has attracted into his life circumstances which allow his world to turn right-side-up again and put him in a placed marked "for winners only." The ultimate outcome of any situation rests in a person's reactions to that situation. In order to discover the born winner in yourself you must learn how to deal with negative thinking whether it occurs only occasionally or has become a habit for you. This chapter will provide you with all the knowledge and methods you need in order to cure any form of negative thinking and find yourself always in the winners' circle.

John A. is a man who learned these facts the hard way. When I first met John, he was working as a plumber for a very large company. He had planned for three years to start his own plumbing business, but, according to John, something always came up and money he saved was needed elsewhere or the deal that looked just perfect fell through. As Mr. A. told me some of the situations which had arisen to cancel out his chance to start his own company, it became clear that he never really believed the day would come when he would own his own plumbing business.

"I stayed optimistic right from the start, even though I always knew I'd never really have my own business. I saved my money, I made my plans, I followed through on the deals and then, just as I knew it would, at the last minute it always fell through."

John was pulling the ground right out from under himself and didn't even realize it. Can you spot the negative attitudes lurking in John's words? Those negative thoughts were enough to keep John exactly where he felt he would always be—working for someone else. As long as John persisted in this way of thinking there was nothing anyone could do to change his situation. He had one big hope and that was to be cured of his negative thinking. His wife, Gladys, finally convinced him that the miracle of metaphysical healing offered him exactly what he needed. With his negative thinking under control for the time being he paid me a visit to inquire about metaphysical healing and a cure of negative thinking.

"Mind you now, I'm not saying that I am a negative thinker. My wife and some of my friends seem to think I am, but as far as I'm concerned I'm only being realistic. Going around smiling like some kind of idiot when I know things aren't going to work out sure isn't going to help matters one bit."

John A.'s control over his negative thinking was slipping right before my eyes and I had to make him hear the negativity which was already creeping into his speech.

"How come you're always so sure things won't work out?"

"It doesn't take any kind of genius to figure that out. After all, things never have worked out, why should they work out now?"

"John, have you ever considered that just by expecting yourself to fail that you are contributing to your own failure? How can you expect other people to believe in you when you don't believe in yourself?"

John's face registered surprise, and it was evident that he was considering these facts for the first time. We talked for an hour and John decided that he would give the miracle of metaphysical healing a chance in his life by using the miraculous techniques of energized mind to break his loser cycle. He agreed to follow the step-by-step method outlined for him and to keep me informed as to his progress in his battle against negative thinking. John had definitely ended our visit on a very positive note.

A phone call from John three weeks after his visit informed me that he was doing much better in general and seemed somehow to be a happier person. He was quick to point out, however, that he had not had any new opportunities to set up his own plumbing business but he truly believed the opportunity would present itself. After one month of silence I heard from John again.

John's voice bubbled from my end of the telephone with such vitality that I was tempted to hold the receiver with both hands. It didn't take ESP to know that something really good had happened to John.

"I did it. I did it today. I signed all the papers and I am now the owner of my own plumbing business. The location is perfect, the lease is perfect, and everything else including the price is just as perfect. I don't doubt one little bit that this business is going to be a winner all the way."

John's voice didn't lose one bit of enthusiasm as he filled me in on the details. He sounded like an entirely different person from the man who had visited me almost two months ago. He was enthusiastic, self-assured, and filled with the certainty that everything was going to turn out 100 percent okay.

"You know, to be truthful with you I thought you were just a little bit off when you told me that the way a person thinks has that much effect on his life. Well, I owe you an apology. You are absolutely correct. For me and my family negative thinking is a poison we don't use and the whole family uses the technique of energized mind to make sure negative thinking stays out of our lives."

John and Gladys A. visited me several months later to tell me that they were opening an additional business location and that things were going just great. With two locations and six plumbers working for him John was already looking forward to the opening of a third location in the very near future. This man has discovered an unbeatable force within himself—the power of energized mind which allows him to remain in touch with the natural born winner he truly is.

The seven miracle steps of energized mind which John A. and thousands of others have used to cure negative thinking and break the loser cycle are presented for you later in this chapter. There is no way this miracle technique can fail to assure you of a 100 percent success in a cure from negative thinking and a happy outcome to all your plans. Before presenting this miracle technique to you, however, I would like to share one more case in which these seven miracle steps were used in order to save an individual from the loser cycle and bring about a cure from the fatal disease of negative thinking.

WOMAN CURES HER SKIN PROBLEMS BY CURING HER NEGATIVE THINKING

Janet B. could easily have won a prize as one of the world's outstanding negative thinkers. Janet did not feel that anything of much good had ever occurred in her life, that anything of much good was now occurring in her life, or that anything of any value would ever occur in her life. Thanks to a lifetime of habitual negative thinking, Janet B. attracted negative circumstances to herself without expending the least bit of effort.

One of the negative circumstances Janet had attracted to herself was a skin condition which manifested itself in a rash which Janet reported itched terribly. She had sought the help of five skin specialists without really ever believing that any one of them could provide the answer to her skin problem. Her negative thinking did not go unrewarded, for her skin disease remained a mystery, not to be treated successfully by any of the five specialists.

"It's no use going to another skin specialist since that one wouldn't be able to find the answer to my problem, either. I'd just be throwing my money away and getting nothing for my time and effort. This is just something I'll have to live with."

It seemed that Janet B. was not the only person in her family who was to live with her skin problem. Five months before Janet visited me, her oldest daughter, who was fifteen, began to suffer the same skin irritation. It showed the same resistance to treatment which it evidenced in Janet's case.

"I told Carol that she'd probably catch the same thing. I also told her that doctors wouldn't be able to treat her either. Well, I was right. We both have to live with this terrible skin disease.

"The next one who will have the same thing is my youngest daughter, Donna."

I was sure that 12 year old Donna could remain untouched by this skin irritation and that Carol's problem would clear up, too, if I could convince Janet B. to use the seven miraculous steps for the cure of negative thinking. Janet protested loudly at first that she had come to see me in order to find the metaphysical healing method that would cure the skin irritation which she and Carol suffered. She felt that I was being ridiculous to offer some metaphysical method for negative thinking when she did not feel herself to be the slightest bit negative in any of her thoughts.

Following an hour and a half discussion Janet finally admitted that negative thinking might play some part in the unfortunate circumstances which turned up constantly in her life. She agreed to carry out the metaphysical healing exercises which would use her energized mind to cure negative thinking. Janet was to keep in touch with me and let me know not only how her skin irritation was, but how her daughter Carol and her daughter Donna were both getting along.

Three weeks later Janet B. was back for another visit, but this time she was minus the skin irritation from which she had suffered on her first visit. It didn't really surprise me that Janet B. looked very different on this visit. She was smiling, her face was free from undue muscle tension, and she seemed to be happy with herself.

"I sure am glad you talked me into trying that technique. My rash is completely gone and so is Carol's. Donna never did develop a rash. That's only part of the story, though.

"Our whole home seems happier. My husband just got a promotion on his job and Carol just got elected to the Student Council in her high school.

"Everything is just better. I feel 100 percent better and I intend to continue using that exercise every single day."

Janet's cure from habitual negative thinking had brought changes to all areas of her life. This is the rule rather than the exception since negative thinking can affect every area of an individual's life. It's nice to know that one exercise of metaphysical healing can bring about a cure from habitual negative thinking and at the same time introduce health and happiness into all areas of a person's life which have been affected by negative thinking.

It is now time that you learn this miracle technique that will banish negativity from your life and the lives of your loved ones. Don't forget the fact that you can use this miraculous technique for the benefit of all negative thinkers for whom you wish to carry out this exercise. This provides you with a very effective means of actually doing something about the negativity in our world today. Don't curse the darkness; instead learn these seven miracle steps of energized mind. Banish the darkness for good and replace it with the natural-born winner that lives within every human being.

YOUR SEVEN MIRACULOUS STEPS FOR THE CURE OF NEGATIVE THINKING

Perform this exercise three times a day for yourself and your loved ones. Remember you need only insert the name of a loved one in order to have that individual benefit from the miraculous healing powers set free by this exercise.

1. Select a location in which you are not likely to be interrupted. Lie down or sit in a chair whose back is high enough to support your head.

2. Close your eyes and for a moment watch the intake and outflow of your breath without any attempt to control it. Allow yourself to become aware of the increased relaxation which is beginning to fill your mind and body.

3. Take a deep breath through your nostrils, being sure to extend your diaphragm as you inhale. Upon completion of inhalation, relax your stomach muscles completely and allow your consciousness to follow the breath, bringing it to rest finally in the area of your head. Repeat this process three times and with each repetition allow your consciousness to be more and more aware of the total relaxation now filling your mind and body.

4. Repeat the following words to yourself mentally: "In the wisdom of my high self and through the power of my energized mind I recognize that I am responsible for my thoughts. I realize that my thoughts are the seeds from which grow all the circumstances of my life and I command my high self to use the power of my energized mind to keep all negativity from my thoughts. My mind on all levels of consciousness will be constantly aware of the fact that my thoughts create that which I experience and will cast out all negativity whether habitual or occasional. Negative thinking shall be alien to me from this moment on."

5. Take a deep breath through your nostrils, extending your diaphragm as you inhale. Upon completion of inhalation com-

pletely relax your stomach muscles and allow your consciousness to follow the breath bringing it to rest finally in the area of
your head. Repeat this process three times and with each repetition allow yourself to be more and more aware of the total
relaxation now filling your body and mind.

6. Repeat the following words to yourself mentally: "In the
wisdom of my high self and through the power of my energized
mind I shall be guarded from all negative thinking, whether
those thoughts are introduced by an individual or a group. The
power of my energized mind shall surround me and I will never
again be affected by the negative thoughts of another."

7. For a moment watch the intake and outflow of your breath
without attempting to control it. Allow yourself to be very aware
of the complete relaxation filling your body and mind. With the
awareness of this relaxation in your consciousness open your
eyes and go about your daily life.

These seven miraculous steps are guaranteed to free you and
your loved ones from negative thinking. If you have been an occasional or habitual negative thinker, it is time that you allow this
miraculous exercise of metaphysical healing to cure you from this
fatal disease. If you have ever watched a loved one suffering from his
or her own negative thoughts, it is time that you introduced the
miracle of metaphysical healing into their life and freed them from
this horrible bondage.

Begin immediately to use these miraculous seven steps in order
to make your life and the lives of your loved ones a monument to
healthy thoughts. Use this technique today to banish negative thinking and bring out the winner in yourself and your loved ones.

THOUGHTS THAT HEAL

You can still enjoy the miracle of metaphysical healing when
your day is so packed with activity that ten seconds of free time seems
an incredible luxury. In times like these use the five miracle thoughts
which are given to you here in order to unlock the power of energized
mind and bring the blessing and comfort of healthy thinking into your
life. In the presence of healthy thoughts even the negative circumstances of confusion and tension must disappear. As little as ten

seconds of your time can bring you comfort and tranquility in the midst of tension and chaos.

Use these miraculous thoughts as often as you wish during the day. The more often you use these miracle thoughts the more strongly does your mind become closed to all negative forms of thought. Learn these miracle thoughts today in order to insure yourself a happier tomorrow.

YOUR FIVE MIRACLE THOUGHTS
THAT CANNOT FAIL TO HEAL

1. "I am a magnificent creation and I share in the creative force which powers this universe."

2. "In each man is the reflection of every man. I am a reflection of the ultimate force which has made all things."

3. "I share the unlimited potential of all creation. My thoughts are the building blocks of my future."

4. "The beauty of my mind is unsurpassed by the loveliness of any sunset. I will not mar the magnificence of my mind with even one negative thought."

5. "My thoughts are the building blocks from which my world is created. In order to fill my world with endless beauty I shall think only beautiful thoughts."

Mentally call to mind one or all five of these miracle thoughts depending on the time available to you. These miraculous thoughts will keep you safe from the negativity in the world and constantly in touch with your own high self and the power of your energized mind.

You need never be the victim of negative thinking again. The knowledge and miracle methods given to you in this chapter will cure you from all negative thinking and keep you safe from the negativity which others place in the world. Begin to use this miraculous technique and these miracle thoughts today in order to banish all negativity and make healthy thinking a habit in your everyday life.

eleven

Metaphysical Healing
Can Cure the Disease of Unhappiness

Are you a person who suffers from chronic unhappiness? Are any of your loved ones sufferers of this terrible self-inflicted disease? If your answer to either or both of these questions is yes, this chapter holds a special benefit for you. In this chapter you will gain the knowledge and learn the miracle methods by which the disease of unhappiness is cured through metaphysical healing and replaced by enjoyment and happiness in your everyday life.

People are not by nature unhappy creatures. Just as our body and mind incline themselves to health so do we as human beings incline ourselves to happiness. It is a cold, hard fact that many people on our planet suffer from unhappiness and that some have suffered for so long that they don't even realize that they are unhappy. Chronic unhappiness often leads to a condition in which its victim is afraid to be happy and in any happy condition seeks for ways which will place the individual once again in unhappy circumstances.

If you have answered yes to either or both of the questions at the beginning of this chapter, can you explain the source of your loved one's or your own unhappiness? Why are you unhappy and what are you willing to do to cure yourself of this disease? The miracle of metaphysical healing and the miraculous techniques you will learn here will enable you to conquer unhappiness and to follow the natural inclination of your own being, which is to enjoy a happy and healthy life.

Do you know why you or a loved one is unhappy? Often people do not find it easy to pinpoint the source of their own unhappiness and thereby add a feeling of vague discomfort to aggravate their already unhappy existence. The miracle technique you are about to learn for the diagnosis of the cause of your own unhappiness can also be used by you to help your loved ones decide the cause of their unhappiness, too. If you are using this miraculous diagnostic method for a loved one, simply present the questions to that individual and then evaluate the answers you receive.

As you zero in on the cause of your own unhappiness it may surprise you to find that at the root of all unhappiness is the individual who is confused concerning goals, values, and the definition of happiness itself. No matter how hard a person tries to blame another for his or her unhappiness the fact remains that it is the individual who sentences himself to this disease, and unless the disease is cured that individual will lead an unappreciated and wasted life.

Use the miraculous technique presented as follows for your loved one or for yourself and discover the cause of unhappiness which threatens to waste the life of another human being.

YOUR MIRACULOUS METHOD OF ENERGIZED MIND FOR THE DIAGNOSIS OF THE CAUSE OF UNHAPPINESS

Be sure to complete each part of this miracle diagnostic technique before reading further into the chapter. Use a pencil and paper to record your answers for each section before proceeding to the next section.

1. Complete the following sentence three times, ending this section with three separate answers.

"I wish . . ."

As you complete the sentence three times the only limitation placed on your wishes is that you may not wish for any additional wishes.

Your paper should now read:

1. I wish (your completion of the sentence).
2. I wish (your completion of the sentence).
3. I wish (your completion of the sentence).

When you have completed this sentence three times you are ready to move to section two.

2. Repeat the following sentence three times without referring to your sentence completions for section one.

"I want . . ."

Your paper should now contain this additional information:

Section Two.

1. I want (your completion of the sentence).
2. I want (your completion of the sentence).
3. I want (your completion of the sentence).

For the moment do not concern yourself with whether wishes and wants are the same things. This will be discussed later in this chapter. Just follow your feelings in completing these sentences.

When you have completed section two you are ready to progress to section three.

3. Complete the following sentence three times without referring to either section one or section two of the work you have already finished.

"I need . . ."

Your paper should contain the following additional information:

Section Three.

1. I need (your completion of the sentence).
2. I need (your completion of the sentence).
3. I need (your completion of the sentence).

When you have completed section three read all your responses over but be sure not to change any of your wording. Now you are ready to evaluate your responses.

Are your answers for sections one and two identical? Do you consider a wish and a want the same thing? You may be surprised to learn that unhappiness can come into a person's life when that individual confuses wishes and wants.

How would you define a wish? Is a wish something you desire very badly? Is a wish something you feel you will never really have? What is your definition of a wish? Take a moment to think about this before reading on in this chapter.

A widely-accepted practical and psychological definition of a wish is a strong desire that is not backed by the energy necessary to attain it. You can see this definition in operation in the following example: From the time I was a child I wished that I could play classical music on the piano. I still wish I could play classical music on a piano, but I have never backed up that wish by taking piano lessons.

When I was a young teenager I wished that I would become a neurosurgeon. I never backed that wish up by applying for medical school or attempting in any way to receive the training that would be necessary to allow me to attain the fulfillment of my wish.

Wishes are clearly strong desires that people do not back up with the energy necessary to bring them into reality. They may seem very important to us, but if we consider the fact that we are not willing to work to fulfill them, their true importance to us begins to be seen in its proper perspective.

What is the true definition of a want? What does it mean to want a certain thing or a certain circumstance in our life? Is a want the same as a wish? Take a moment now to consider these questions in your own mind before continuing with this chapter.

A widely-accepted practical and psychological definition of a want is a strong desire backed by whatever energy is necessary to attain that desire. This definition is made more clear for you in the following example. I decided when I was in high school that I wanted to go to college. I backed up this want by taking a college preparatory course during my high school years and then making formal application to a university. Since I also wanted to graduate from college, I took the necessary required courses at the university and the necessary number of electives in order to complete the requirements for graduation. Unlike my desire to play classical music on a piano which, for me, was only a wish, my desire to attend and graduate from college was a strong want backed by energy in the form of action that was designed to bring what I wanted into reality.

Read your wishes and wants over again and think about them for a few moments. Are your three listings of wants truly desires which you are willing to back with energy and action? If your answer is no then you cannot stop deluding yourself any longer, and admit to yourself that you may wish for these things but truly do not want them in your life. What individual would be so foolish as to be unhappy at the absence of something or some circumstance in his life which he really didn't want there anyway? Have you spent time being unhappy because you did not have a thing or circumstance which you truly didn't want in the first place?

You may now look at your responses to section three. What is a need? Is a need something you want very strongly and are willing to put all the action necessary behind it in order to achieve its reality? Is a need anything like a wish? Do you feel that your needs are as numerous as your wishes and wants? Take the time to consider these questions for a moment in your own mind.

A need has been widely-defined practically and psychologically as a thing or circumstance necessary to the existence of a person's "self." This, too, will become more clear as you read the following example. I truly need very few things and circumstances in my life. I need, as all human beings do, food, shelter, clothing, security, and a feeling that I am worthwhile. I need to love and to be loved. I do not need $1,000,000. It would be possible for me at this time to wish for or even want $1,000,000, but it would be untrue to say that I actually needed $1,000,000 in my life as it is now. Unless you have $1,000,000 worth of debts and/or expenses in your life, you cannot truly say that you have need of this amount of money at this time in your life. This is not to say that you may not wish for or even want $1,000,000 by backing your strong desire for this amount of money with actions that are designed to bring your desire into actuality.

It often happens that unhappiness is brought into an individual's life by confusing wishes and wants with needs. Sometimes people feel they need much more than they actually do in order to fulfill the "self" in them. Many individuals make themselves unhappy by screaming that their needs are not being met and not realizing that their complaints are not legitimate ones. Don't allow such confusions to introduce unhappiness to you. Take the time now to give some serious thoughts to your needs. Have you been complaining about unfulfilled needs that weren't really needs at all? Have you been unhappy because none of your wishes seemed to come true? Realize now that wishes are not backed by the stuff that will make them a reality. If you have been unhappy because the things you want have not fallen into your lap, know now that you must put the energy and effort behind these strong desires in order to have them take the shape of realities in your life.

If you have spent much of your time being unhappy concerning things and events which confused you from the start, decide now not to spend another moment of your time in useless unhappiness. Stop crying about things you never really wanted or needed. Enjoy your wishes but realize that unless you are willing to turn those wishes into wants, you don't really desire the wished for things or events in your life. Surely you would not be so foolish as to spend time in unhappiness over things you never really wanted anyway.

No matter where you placed the blame for your unhappiness

before, you can now use this miraculous diagnostic technique in order to find the true cause of your unhappiness. Once you have taken this step you will be ready to use the miraculous technique of metaphysical healing for the cure of all unhappiness.

MAN CURES HIS CHRONIC UNHAPPINESS THROUGH THE MIRACLE OF METAPHYSICAL HEALING

If anyone decided to offer a prize to the unhappiest person alive, David R. would surely have won first prize. David was 30 when I met him and owned a bakery in partnership with his father. From what David told me, both men were very unhappy, but if they were being ranked for prizes David still would have taken first place. If anyone had asked David what had made him unhappy enough to win first prize in an unhappiness contest, he would not have been able to tell you. David truthfully did not know the cause of his own unhappiness.

"I can't figure it out myself. My business is doing great, I've been married for eight years and have a lovely wife and two great children, but still I'm very unhappy. I realize how quickly all the things for which I should be happy could be taken away from me and then I can't be happy even though I have those things now. It's strange, but my father seems to be the only one who understands what I'm talking about when I tell people why I'm unhappy.

"My wife has been down in the mouth now for almost a year and my two children are beginning to show the same signs of unhappiness that I feel, and believe me that worries me quite a bit. I don't want my family to be unhappy and if I'm causing that unhappiness I want to get rid of whatever I'm doing to make myself unhappy."

"Mr. R., do you realize what you just said? You said that if you are making your family unhappy you want to get rid of whatever is causing your unhappiness. Wouldn't you like to get rid of your unhappiness simply because it makes you unhappy?"

"I didn't even realize I said that. Of course I want to get rid of my own unhappiness just for myself, too. My family, though, my family is real important to me and I don't want my family unhappy.

"If I knew why I was unhappy and how to change it I would have changed it already. I wouldn't be here talking to you if I already knew those things, believe me. I'm here because I heard about this metaphysical healing stuff and I want to learn how to cure my own unhappiness. Now Jimmy, my friend, has explained to me that you have some kind of technique that will allow me to find out why I'm really unhappy first and then you have another method that allows me to get rid of this unhappiness from myself.

"I want you to teach me that—what do you call it?— metaphysical healing to get rid of unhappiness."

We spent some time talking about David's father and it became clear that unhappiness was a common ailment in David's whole family. It was as if David had caught the disease from his father and was now about to transmit it to his own children.

"Well, what good will it do for me to be cured if my father still suffers from what do you call this disease of unhappiness? Can we cure him at the same time?"

I assured David that the same metaphysical healing technique which was guaranteed to work for him would also work for his father. David agreed to give the miracle diagnostic technique for the true cause of unhappiness to his father and, as David put it, "talk him into using metaphysical healing for himself." When David had completed this technique himself his answers showed that one of the main reasons for David's unhappiness was that he was confusing his wants with what he felt people thought he should want. For example, people had been telling David for quite a while that he needed to expand the business. David knew that that was one way to indicate that a business was making progress, but for some reason, whenever an opportunity arose for the bakery to expand either David or his father became ill and the plans had to be canceled. As we talked it became clear that David really did not want to expand his business at all, but was very content with the size of the business at present. Although his father agreed that expansion was a great idea I was willing to bet that if David gave him the diagnostic technique his father, too, would find that he was very happy with business the way it was and had no desire for expansion.

"Now that's something else. I would have bet anything in the world that I wanted to expand that business. Now I can see that I am really happy with the way things are; I don't want the bakery to be any bigger. I guess I just wanted to want what people felt I should want."

After we discussed the metaphysical healing technique to cure the disease of unhappiness David left with a promise to contact me in the future. He had agreed to do quite a bit more thinking about his responses to the miracle diagnostic technique for the true cause of unhappiness.

It was two months before I saw David again and when he paid me the second visit he came bearing gifts. He had brought a box of donuts which he had baked, a quart of milk, and a package of paper cups.

"I just thought you might enjoy having a snack while I told you about what's been happening in the last two months."

David opened the box of donuts and I poured us both a paper cup of cold milk. As we relaxed and enjoyed the donuts from his bakery, David began to fill me in on what had happened since I last saw him.

"Actually, I could have been back to see you in three weeks. I decided to wait until Pop got cured, too. You see it took him a little longer because it took me longer to talk him into taking the diagnostic technique for what's causing unhappiness. If I had been a better salesman I would have been visiting you again a lot sooner.

"I did a lot of thinking about my answers to that technique and I really decided that I wasn't as unhappy as I thought I was. I was making myself unhappy by trying to fit other people's ideas of what I should have and what I should give my wife and my children and what I should do with my spare time. Well, I don't worry about any of that anymore. In fact, I really don't worry anymore period. I used that miracle method for the cure of unhappiness and believe me I'm cured and my family would be the first to tell you so."

David paused for a moment and took a long drink of milk and then continued.

"Pop is cured, too. I wish you could see—I mean the change in him. He's like a new person. Neither one of us worries about losing the things that make us happy anymore and we both discovered that we're perfectly happy with our business which is doing great and, if I do say so myself, is the best bakery in town.

"My wife is happier because I'm happier and my kids are no longer showing signs of becoming old before their time. They are really happy kids. Everything is fantastic and, if you haven't guessed it by now, I am a very happy man."

I had guessed the fact that David was happy. With the smile on his face, the enthusiasm in his voice, and the light that seemed to shine from his eyes it didn't take a genius to figure that fact out. The miracle of metaphysical healing had completely changed David R.'s life and had also cured his father from chronic unhappiness. It was not surprising to hear that David's family was enjoying the benefits of David's cure from unhappiness. Happiness is not a disease, but it is just as contagious as unhappiness.

The same miraculous metaphysical technique which healed David of his unhappiness will also work for you and those you love. Why spend another day of your life unhappy or watch a loved one waste time in unhappiness? The metaphysical healing technique which is presented for your benefit in this chapter is guaranteed to cure unhappiness no matter what its cause happens to be. Join the thousands of people who have already discovered that this miraculous healing method cures unhappiness and restores the natural balance of unhappiness which is inherent in your nature itself. I seem to remember an old saying that goes "the Lord loves a cheerful giver." That may very well be a fact but I would like to paraphrase that saying so that it states another truth. "The Creator loves a cheerful liver."

YOUR SEVEN MIRACLE STEPS TO HAPPINESS

If you use these seven miraculous steps of metaphysical healing for a loved one simply insert that loved one's name in the appropriate places.

1. Select a location where you are not likely to be interrupted. Lie down or sit in a chair whose back is high enough to support your head.

2. Take a deep breath through your nostrils, extending your diaphragm as you inhale. Upon completion of inhalation completely relax your stomach muscles and follow the breath through your body, bringing it to rest finally in the area of your head. Repeat this process three times and with each repetition allow yourself to be more and more aware of the total relaxation which now begins to fill your body and mind.

3. Repeat the following words to yourself mentally: "In the wisdom of my high self and through the power of my energized mind I recognize the splendor that surrounds me in my everyday living. Several times each day happy memories shall be brought into my consciousness and I shall recognize and appreciate the happiness which has filled my life in the past, is filling my life now, and will continue to fill my life in the future."

4. Allow your consciousness to be aware of the intake and out-flow of your breath without attempting to control it. Allow yourself to be more and more aware of the total relaxation now filling your body and mind.

5. Repeat the following words to yourself mentally: "'I in my humanness am the most precious part of all creation. Through the wisdom of my high self and by the power of my energized mind I shall see life and enjoy it through the magnificence which is inherent within myself. I shall look through eyes which see beauty in all that surrounds me, whether that beauty is reflected in a beautiful painting or a single daffodil in a field. Through my ears I shall hear beauty in all sounds that break this world's silence, and in that silence itself I shall hear an even deeper beauty than can be found in spoken sounds. I shall thrill to the beauty of textures that surround me whether I am touching the most expensive velvet or the lush textures of grasses that bend beneath my touch and then spring back to add their beauty to the created world.

"My life shall be one grand song in which I sing in my heart in appreciation for the beauty with which I have been surrounded and the precious gift of life which enables me to appreciate that beauty. Although I may never own one forest or an ocean or a sky filled with bubbles of lacy clouds I shall have them all for my own in that I will appreciate them fully."

6. Recall the faces of several of your loved ones and repeat the following words to yourself mentally: "For all who have loved me and whom I have loved I am thankful. For all people who have cared about my welfare at any time in my life and who have taken time from their lives to think of me I am grateful. My appreciation and happiness shall swell out and touch all with whom I come into contact, enriching their lives and mine a hundredfold."

7. Repeat the following words to yourself mentally: "Each day shall find me more understanding and appreciative of the gift of life. My appreciation shall increase my happiness, and my happiness shall increase my appreciation. I shall come to know more and more every day a true set of values in my heart and mind and never again will I judge myself by another man's measuring stick. I shall never waste time on trifles but will find much happiness in little things. From this place in time onward I

shall be aware of my own magnificence and of the magnificence of creation which surrounds me. I shall be filled with the happiness of this creation and never again waste one moment in unhappiness or sorrow.''

Open your eyes and go about your daily life.

These seven miraculous steps are guaranteed to cure you and your loved ones from the disease of unhappiness which can make your life miserable and add misery to the lives of those around you. There is no way this miraculous technique can fail to restore you to happiness since the miracle of metaphysical healing knows no limitations and is backed by the power of your energized mind which knows a force that knows no limits.

Don't waste another moment of your time. Begin to use this seven step miraculous method today in order to insure happiness for yourself and all you love.

HOW TO DEAL WITH UNHAPPINESS IN OTHERS

Recall to memory a time when you felt discomfort at not knowing what to do or say in the presence of unhappiness in a loved one. That feeling of helplessness can lead to discomfort in many situations, but thanks to the miracle of metaphysical healing you are never helpless to deal with unhappiness in anyone. No matter what the cause of unhappiness in those you love, the miracle of metaphysical healing gives you the ability to restore each of your loved ones to a sense of well-being in happiness.

You can accomplish this without spending a great deal of time talking to loved ones and explaining to them the fact that they really have much more reason to be happy than to be unhappy. In fact, in order to bring a smile to the faces of those you love, you need not speak even one word to them. Your own happiness and appreciation of life will naturally radiate to all with whom you come into contact and, in many respects, will be contagious for them. What could be nicer to catch than a good case of happiness?

The simple but miraculous technique which follows will allow you to make your happiness more contagious to all those you love. It will amplify your own happiness and send it into the hearts of everyone around you, allowing them to discover their own happiness in themselves. It is a miracle technique which works quickly and with no possibility of failure in allowing everyone around you to recognize and attain the happiness which is their birthright. You can use this technique for as many individuals at one time as you wish. You can use this miraculous technique in a crowded room or any place you happen to meet people who are unhappy.

Begin today to share your happiness with others and you will find that your own happiness will also increase.

YOUR MIRACLE OF METAPHYSICAL HEALING THAT WILL BRING A SMILE TO ANYONE'S FACE

1. Repeat the following words to yourself mentally: "In the wisdom of my high self and through the power of my energized mind I will that all those around me will be relieved of their unhappiness and filled with the happiness and joy which is theirs through their birthright. I will that smiles replace frowns and tears of joy replace tears of sorrow."

2. Recall in your own mind one aspect of the created world which you appreciate and spend a moment enjoying your appreciation of that aspect.

Repeat the following words to yourself mentally: "I will that the joy and happiness I feel shall now overflow and touch the hearts of all around me."

This miraculous technique is guaranteed to relieve the unhappiness of those around you and replace their frowns with smiles. Later on, when it is possible, you may wish to perform the seven miracle steps for the cure of unhappiness for these individuals. The miraculous technique which has just been given to you is extremely useful in emergency situations and in circumstances when you do not have the privacy or the time to carry out the seven miracle steps of metaphysical healing for the cure of unhappiness. There is no way in which this miraculous technique or any of the miracle methods of metaphysical healing presented for your benefit in this book can fail you.

The more you use the miraculous techniques presented for you in this chapter, the more alien will unhappiness become in your life and the lives of your loved ones. If you but follow the seven miracle steps for the cure of unhappiness you will find that happiness becomes an everyday condition in your everyday life. Start today to use this miraculous technique and make unhappiness a thing of the past and fill your life with the joy that is your birthright.

twelve

How to Form a Metaphysical Healing Group

Although the old saying, "Two heads are better than one," contains some truth, there are many areas in life where an individual must work out his or her problems without the aid of another human being. In the field of metaphysical healing, "Two heads can often be better than one." The miraculous power of energized mind which allows the miracle of metaphysical healing to take place can in some respects be compared to a battery. When more than one individual focuses the power of energized mind and directs it for a single purpose the force of that power can be greatly enhanced.

The metaphysical healing group offers people the opportunity to join with fellow human beings for the purpose of directing the concentrated force of energized mind to bring the miracle of metaphysical healing into reality. You are well-aware that in many jobs where great force and strength is needed, the addition of another individual to the work crew can make the job lighter for all concerned and shorten the time it will take to complete that job. The metaphysical healing group offers these two advantages in addition to others which will be discussed later in this chapter to the people who take part in its activities.

You will understand these two advantages even more clearly if you allow yourself to consider the great force and power possessed by a laser beam. You are well-acquainted with the light which can fill a room at the flick of a switch. As the switch is turned electricity surges through wiring and a light bulb fills the room with diffused light. Diffused light spreads over the entire room so that it does not appear as a beam of light but rather an overall presence of light. In contrast to diffused light which can fill a room, many lasers use a form of compacted light which takes the shape of a beam and has the power to cut a bar of steel in half. The amazing power of this laser beam has in principle much in common with a metaphysical healing group. The metaphysical healing group combines and compacts the miraculous power of many energized minds and directs it toward a single purpose. In joining and forming such a healing group you will find that, as in the case of the addition of another worker on any job, you will find your work load lightened and the time it takes to complete your task shortened.

In addition to the advantages mentioned above, there are other important advantages which you will derive from the formation of and participation in a metaphysical healing group. One advantage which you will discover very quickly is the help you yourself can obtain from the other members of the group in regard to your own health matters and the health matters of your loved ones and in an exchange of information concerning the miracle of metaphysical healing. Your group can create a life line for the flow of energized mind directing the miracle of metaphysical healing to all whose names are presented to the group and to the group members themselves.

In emergency situations this life line for the flow of energized mind can be used by the group for a metaphysical healing hot line which in a matter of moments can have all group members sending the miracle of metaphysical healing to an individual or people anywhere in the world in need of emergency metaphysical healing. This same healing hot line will stand ready to serve you and your loved ones whenever and wherever that help is needed. Blood banks which guarantee you and your loved ones life-giving blood in emergency situations can give you comfort with the guarantee that if and when you and your loved ones are in need of a transfusion the blood needed will be there. Your metaphysical healing hot line offers you an even greater amount of comfort with the assurance that you and your loved ones will receive the miracle of metaphysical healing if, when, and where that miraculous power is needed. Your active participation in a metaphysical healing group provides you and your loved ones with a security no ordinary insurance plan can offer. Your active participation in the metaphysical healing group also allows you to express your concern for those you love by making sure that they will always have available to them the unlimited power of energized mind and the miracle of metaphysical healing. Surely you cannot deny this wonderful blessing to your loved ones or yourself.

MIRACLE STEPS TO FOLLOW IN THE FORMATION OF A METAPHYSICAL HEALING GROUP

1. Decide the purpose for which your metaphysical healing group will operate. Will it operate in sending the miracle of metaphysical healing only to group members and their loved ones, or will it be open to requests for the miracle of metaphysical healing from those who may have heard of its work but are not connected with any member specifically?

2. Decide on the optimum number of members you would like in your group. Upper limits of metaphysical healing groups usually reach ten or at the most 15 members, but you must decide whether you wish the number of members to be kept smaller than this number or to be allowed to grow beyond this number in membership.

3. Decide when, where, and how frequently your group will meet. Decide also on the length of each meeting.

Generally, metaphysical healing groups meet once a week, alternately at members' homes, and meetings last on the average of one and one half to two hours. You and the other members of your group can decide what arrangements work best for your group.

4. Decide where your membership will come from. You may already have several friends who have expressed an interest in the miracle of metaphysical healing. If this is so you might wish to ask these friends if they would be interested in participating in a metaphysical healing group.

If you have not discussed this subject previously with your friends, you might wish to introduce the subject of a metaphysical healing group to several of your close friends and ask if they would be interested in joining a metaphysical healing group. It would be wise not to attempt to persuade a person to join your metaphysical healing group if this person has expressed an attitude against belonging to such a group or has shown much hesitation and uncertainty as to whether membership in such a group would interest them. You will find that the type of dedication that will help to make your group successful will be found in members who will willingly welcome the opportunity to participate actively in a metaphysical healing group. Do not be in the least bit concerned if the membership of your group grows slowly. Remember that quantity alone cannot make for a successful group but quality of determination cannot fail but lead to success.

5. Determine to keep accurate records of all cases in which your metaphysical healing group has sent the miracle of metaphysical healing to any individual. Whenever an apparent cure has taken place, get as much documentation of that cure as is possible. This documentation should come from the individual or individuals cured, friends and relatives of that individual or individuals, and, most importantly, from the attending physician if this is at all possible.

6. Obtain as much information as possible concerning the individual to whom metaphysical healing is to be directed. If necessary speak with the physician or consult a medical encyclopedia in order that someone may make clear to all group members the actual physical or mental condition which is to be corrected and cured through the miracle of metaphysical healing.

7. Choose a group leader who will lead the metaphysical healing group in the appropriate miraculous techniques of energized mind and ultra-mind in order to direct the miracle of metaphysical healing. You may wish to alternate group leadership so that each member will have the opportunity to become fully acquainted with leading the miraculous techniques of metaphysical healing.

8. Determine whether your group will work exclusively with medical and mental illness, disease, and injury, or will also include the direction of metaphysical healing for the cure of financial illness and injury and the cure of injured and broken relationships. Both these situations can be cured through the miracle of metaphysical healing and both are legitimate concerns for the metaphysical healing group. It is entirely a matter of group preference as to whether your group will deal with these problems.

9. Do not allow your group meetings to become strictly social affairs. Coffee, tea, soft drinks, and conversation following a meeting is fine as long as this activity remains secondary to the primary purpose for the meeting which is the use of energized mind and ultra-mind to direct the miracle of metaphysical healing. Most groups have at one time or another experienced a problem along this line, so keep your eyes open and if the problem does arise remind the group members of the purposes and goals of your group in order that the problem should not get out of hand.

10. Decide that all members of your group will be honor-bound not to discuss personal information concerning individuals who come to your attention because they are seeking the miracle of metaphysical healing. Seek always to help, stoop never to judge.

11. Set up a healing hot line in your group. This metaphysical healing hot line will be used in all cases of emergency situations. In order to guarantee its success each member of your group will have the phone numbers of all other members of the group. The member in need of help or who is aware of a group member or a loved one who is in such need will call one group member and explain the situation to him or her. This member will then call one additional member and this process will continue until the entire group has been notified of the emergency situation and is following the miraculous techniques for metaphysical healing in emergency situations as outlined in this book. Make sure that each member knows exactly who he or she is responsible for calling in the case of an emergency where the metaphysical healing hot line is to be used.

With the steps thus presented for you in this chapter and the miracle techniques of metaphysical healing presented for you in this book, you and your group cannot help but be successful in directing the miracle of metaphysical healing and introducing the gift of perfect health and happiness to those in need. Remember that whatever metaphysical healing your group sends out will return to each individual member of your group a thousandfold.

This book provides you and any metaphysical healing group with specific instructions and miraculous techniques for the formation of a healing group and the cure of illness, disease, and injury through the miracle of metaphysical healing. Become well-acquainted with the miraculous techniques provided for you here, so that in the face of illness, injury, or an emergency you will know exactly what miracle technique is needed and how to use its unlimited power. Make this book an important part of your life so that the miraculous techniques included here will place the unlimited power of your energized mind and ultra-mind constantly at your disposal.

thirteen

How to Use the Miracle of Metaphysical Healing to Cure Your Money Problems

Do you or any of your loved ones suffer from financial problems? The power of energized mind stands ready to bring the miracle of metaphysical healing to all your financial illnesses. A sick financial situation can often lead through the path of worry into physical, mental, and emotional illness. You can use the miracle of metaphysical healing to cure all your money problems and attract financial benefits to yourself and those you love.

If you have spent as much as five minutes in your life worrying about bills, this chapter is especially for you. The unlimited power of your energized mind can be used not only to heal financial illness, but can also attract all manner of financial blessings into your life. You need never worry again about meeting your bills. Worrying has never paid a bill yet, but the miracle of metaphysical healing through the power of energized mind has provided millions of people with cures for their financial worries and the power to attract financial benefits into their life. In this chapter you will learn how to use the miracle of metaphysical healing to solve all your money problems and attract into your life all the financial benefits you want. Learn these miraculous techniques now and discover how the power of energized mind can make your thoughts as good as gold.

WOMAN USES THE MIRACLE OF METAPHYSICAL HEALING TO PAY FOR HER HOME

Martha B. had been a widow for two years when I met her. Martha's husband, James, had been killed in an automobile accident in 1971, leaving Martha alone to raise their four year old son, Jimmy. When James died he was only 26 years old and Martha 24. James had worked very hard as an automobile mechanic to provide his family with the necessities of life, but had not bothered to provide more than minimal burial insurance for himself.

"James didn't believe in insurance or in saving money for that matter. He figured we were both young and had a long time ahead of us.

"Don't get me wrong—James was a great husband and father—he just didn't feel that savings and insurance were necessary. He would never deliberately have left Jimmy and me in this position financially."

Martha went on to say that she and her husband had purchased a small home just before his death. The mortgage payments had been no problem since Martha worked as a clerk/typist and James made very good money as a mechanic. Since her husband's death, however, Martha had all she could do to meet her house payment and provide the necessities for herself and her son. Martha had received several small raises in salary on her job, but the cost of living had also increased canceling out the extra benefit those raises might have introduced for Martha and Jimmy.

"What I really need is a really good raise or a new job. I'm already behind one house payment and I'm afraid that if things keep going the way they have been Jimmy and I will lose our home.

"I've taken secretarial courses and I'm very good at shorthand, typing, and composing letters. I feel that I deserve a promotion but so far my company hasn't thought so.

"I want you to teach me to use my energized mind in order to get that promotion along with a substantial increase in salary. That way I won't have to worry about the house payments and, in fact, maybe I can double up on them and Jimmy and I can have our home paid for in no time at all.

"Gail S. told me that you taught her how to use this energized mind thing and she's doing really great financially now. Teach me to use the same thing so that I can get rid of my money problems and get what Jimmy and I need in our lives."

We talked about the miracle of metaphysical healing for financial problems and how to use the power of energized mind to attract financial blessings into one's life. Martha was very determined to use the miraculous techniques daily and promised to let me know how things were going for her and Jimmy. She left with the remark, "When I get my promotion I'll buy you the biggest steak in town."

"Make that an ice cream soda, Martha, and you've got a deal."

About two months later Martha telephoned me. "I just wanted to make sure that you were there. Don't leave, I'll be right over."

Twenty-five minutes later Martha B. walked in carrying a paper bag. "Here's the ice cream soda I owe you. It even has an extra scoop of ice cream.

"I waited to contact you again until I got my first paycheck for my new job. You are now looking at the private secretary to the vice-president of the firm. I got a $400 a month raise and a job that's three times as interesting as what I was doing before.

"No one, including me, thought the woman who had that job would ever quit. As it turned out she quit for a very happy reason. She and her husband have been trying to have a baby for about five years without any success. Well, she's pregnant and she couldn't be happier. She gave her notice as soon as she found out and she recommended me to replace her. I never would have thought she paid the least bit of attention to my work. Anyway, everything turned out great. She and her husband couldn't be happier and neither could I.

"The miracle of metaphysical healing gets an A+ in my books. Thanks an awful lot for teaching me those miraculous techniques.

"Holy cow, I almost forgot. My company credit union has taken over the mortgage for my house and the payments and interest are less than what they were with the bank. It will be a cinch paying for the house now. You might say that the miracle of metaphysical healing is actually buying the house for me and Jimmy."

The same miraculous technique of metaphysical healing which cured the financial problems of Martha B. will also work for you. Start today to heal your money problems by using the power of your energized mind to bring the miracle of metaphysical healing to all your financial woes.

YOUR METAPHYSICAL HEALING TECHNIQUE FOR THE CURE OF FINANCIAL PROBLEMS

Follow this miraculous failproof technique three times a day. It is guaranteed to bring a cure to you and your loved ones for all financial problems

1. Select a location where you are not likely to be interrupted. Lie down or sit in a chair whose back is high enough to support your head.

2. Close your eyes and allow your consciousness to be totally aware of your intake and outflow of breath without attempting to control it. Become completely aware of the new relaxation beginning to flow through your mind and body.

3. Take a deep breath through your nostrils, extending your diaphragm as you inhale. Upon completion of inhalation relax your stomach muscles completely and allow your consciousness to follow your breath throughout your body, bringing it to rest finally in the area of your head. Repeat this process three times and with each repetition allow yourself to be more and more aware of the total relaxation now flowing throughout your body and mind.

4. Repeat the following words to yourself mentally: "Through the power of my energized mind, the miracle of metaphysical healing is now curing all financial ills in my life. Unlimited resources are at the disposal of my energized mind and I now claim all the financial resources necessary to allow me and my family to live comfortably without financial worry. Through the miracle of metaphysical healing I shall never know financial want again."

5. Take a deep breath through your nostrils, extending the diaphragm as you inhale. Upon completion of inhalation, completely relax your stomach muscles and allow your consciousness to follow your breath, bringing it to rest finally in the area of your head. Repeat this process three times and with each repetition allow yourself to be totally aware of the complete relaxation now filling your mind and body.

6. For a moment allow your consciousness to be totally aware of your intake and outflow of breath without attempting to control it. Be totally aware of the complete relaxation which fills your body and mind.

7. Open your eyes and go about your daily life.

You may use this miraculous technique not only for yourself but also for your loved ones simply by inserting your loved one's name in the appropriate places. Don't waste another moment of your life worrying about money problems. This miraculous technique of metaphysical healing will cure your money problems and make them only dim memories of the past.

Through the use of this miraculous technique, the miracle of metaphysical healing will fill your life with opportunities for the legitimate and healthy acquisition of money needed to make you financially secure. This is not to say that money will fall from the heavens into your lap, for such a statement would be ridiculous and an insult to your intelligence. The miracle of metaphysical healing will provide you with all the money you need to cure your financial woes by placing you in a healthy and legitimate position to earn that money or through the creation of circumstances by which you become the happy recipient of an unexpected financial gift or windfall. Money which comes to you through the miracle of metaphysical healing will always have a legitimate and happy source. Start using this miraculous technique today and say good-bye to your money problems.

THE MIRACLE OF METAPHYSICAL HEALING CAN BE USED FOR LUXURIES AS WELL AS NECESSITIES

The miracle of metaphysical healing does not limit you to the bare necessities of life, but will allow you to attract many financial blessings and luxuries into your life. It will allow you to have the things you want when you want them, but it is very important that you know what you want. You would be wise to reread the section in Chapter eleven which provides you with a miraculous technique for determining what it is that you really want in your life. By taking the time to reread this section of Chapter eleven you can be sure that your desires are wants and not merely wishes.

Once you have decided that your desire is a true want, you can use the miraculous technique provided for you in this chapter for the cure of your financial problems and simply add the following paragraph to step four of your metaphysical healing technique for the cure of your financial problems.

"Through the power of my energized mind and through the wisdom of my high self I will also to receive into my life through happy and legitimate means the following luxuries: (here name the luxuries that you want in your life)."

Once you have added this paragraph to step four of your miracle technique, simply continue the remaining three steps of this miraculous failproof method for the cure of your money problems.

MAN USES METAPHYSICAL HEALING
TO GAIN A LUXURY ITEM

Charles K. had used the miracle of metaphysical healing to bring a cure to all his money problems.

"Things are really going great and I really have no complaints about money. What I'm calling you about is that I would like to have a new car. I know I don't really need a new car, but I do want a new car. You mentioned once before that the miracle of metaphysical healing can also be used to obtain luxury items that you really want and I'd like you to teach me the additional steps I have to take in order to use metaphysical healing for this purpose."

I explained to Charles that he could add one paragraph to step four of the miraculous technique he had already used successfully to cure his money problems and through this addition he could obtain the new car which he wanted. Since Charles K. had already experienced the miraculous power of metaphysical healing in putting an end to all his money worries, he was more than anxious to use this additional step in order to obtain his new car.

It was only two weeks later when Charles called me again on the telephone in order to say, "Would you like to see my new car? That's right, I got my new car. That doesn't really come as a surprise to you though, does it?

"Anyway, I just wanted to say thank you for teaching me that additional step and let you know that my whole family is happy with the new car.

"The money came through an unexpected raise at the factory. The pay raise I got will pay the car payments each month.

"Thanks again for letting me in on the miracle of metaphysical healing."

The extra paragraph which Charles K. used to obtain his new car is the same paragraph presented for you here in this chapter. Simply add this new paragraph to step four as you were directed previously and you can use the miracle of metaphysical healing to obtain any luxury which you want in life. Just make sure that the luxury you ask for is something you truly want since this technique cannot fail to bring that which you want into actualization.

If you have any doubts concerning the difference between a wish, a want, and a need reread the section of Chapter eleven which makes these distinctions perfectly clear before you use this additional miraculous step. The addition of this miracle step will allow the miracle of metaphysical healing to bring compound interest into your daily life. In addition to using this miraculous extra step to bring any luxury you want into your life, you may also use this step to heal an unhealthy bank account. Through adding this additional step to your metaphysical healing technique for the cure of money problems you can bring additional money into your life which can be added to your bank account with no financial sacrifice to you or your family.

This miraculous technique of metaphysical healing provides you with your own personal miracle method for complete financial health and security. Begin using your personal miracle today in order to bring financial security into your own life and into the lives of those you love.

fourteen

How to Cure
a Broken Relationship
Through Metaphysical Healing

It's a safe bet that at least once in your life you have experienced the pain of a broken relationship. No one who has experienced the loss of a close relationship can deny that the pain that follows such a loss can be worse than physical torment. There is no non-prescription or prescription drug available today that can offer a cure for such pain or for its cause. The miracle of metaphysical healing offers you both a cure for the pain and a cure for its cause.

There are many books available concerning the social sicknesses which affect our society. One of the main illnesses prevalent in our world today is the decay of the institution of marriage and the family. There are few, if any, psychiatrists and psychologists who would deny that a feeling of not belonging and lack of commitment in relationships has sickened the very roots of our society. These same psychological experts also agree that they can offer no guaranteed short-term cures at present. The institutions of marriage and the family are dying before our eyes of a fatal sickness and the traditional medical world offers us little or no hope for their cure.

Through the power of your energized mind the miracle of metaphysical healing extends to you a guaranteed cure for sick and broken relationships not only for yourself, but for your loved ones as well. The miraculous techniques presented to you in this chapter will allow you to bring the blessing of metaphysical healing to sick and broken relationships which are based on the caring involved in friendship, business, family ties, or marriage. Whether you use these miraculous techniques for yourself or those you love they cannot fail to bring perfect health for any relationship to which you direct the miraculous power of metaphysical healing. You have the power to do today what traditional medicine only hopes to be able to do in the future—cure the broken relationship. Don't waste this precious gift. If your loved ones are in pain due to broken friendships, family ties, or marriages, cure their pain and restore health to their relationships now by starting today to direct the miraculous power of metaphysical healing to them.

HUSBAND AND WIFE USE THE MIRACLE OF ENERGIZED MIND TO HEAL AND REBUILD THEIR MARRIAGE

When Mike and Eilene D. came to see me they were not seeking a traditional marriage counselor. The unhappy couple had spent thousands of dollars and almost one year of their lives seeking a cure for the illness that was killing their relationship and which seemed destined to deliver the fatal blow to their marriage.

"During the past year Mike and I have been to one psychiatrist, one psychologist, and one marriage counselor. None of them have been able to help us put our marriage back together. It's as if our relationship is dying right before our eyes and as much as we want it healed no one knows the cure."

Eilene's face showed her concern as she spoke and Mike's eyes watched her intently reflecting the same sincere concern about their dying marriage.

"The real trouble started when I got a promotion and had to spend quite a bit of time out of town. I have to admit that Eilene was really good about it at first, but when it looked like it was going to be a regular thing she began to lose patience fast. I guess she got lonely and I can't blame her for that.

"About a year ago she decided that she wanted a divorce. We talked about our commitment to marriage and our love for each other and decided to seek professional help. It took me six months to find a job where I didn't have to travel and that six months was costly to both of us. I was out of town more than I was home and Eilene grew constantly more disenchanted with me and the whole idea of being married to me. Now that I'm home the problem has been getting to know each other again and seeing if we can both recapture the in love feelings that were there before. Psychological help has not done much to help our situation and when Eilene's sister told us about metaphysical healing for marriage problems we decided to come speak with you. We really want our marriage to work and we'd like you to teach us this metaphysical healing technique in order to cure our marriage problems and make our relationship a healthy one again.''

We talked for about an hour and I explained to Mike and Eilene the metaphysical healing technique for the cure of an unhealthy or dying marriage. They were both eager to begin using the miraculous technique immediately and said they would keep me posted on the results.

Three months later I received a phone call from Mike, and his happiness was contagious even over the telephone.

"Things are working out great. Eilene and I have never been happier. In fact, we just found out this week that Eilene is going to have a baby. Isn't that great?

"I'd say we'd name the kid after you if it was a girl but to be honest with you I can't stand the name Evelyn. We both want you to know, though, that we're very grateful that you taught us how to use metaphysical healing to cure the sickness in our marriage. Our kid will learn about metaphysical healing as soon as he is old enough to understand. If you hadn't guessed, I'm hoping for a boy.

"Thanks again for everything. Eilene and I will keep in touch."

Seven and one half months later I received a birth announcement informing me that Michael Richard D. had arrived on schedule and in addition to being the cutest baby ever born was also 100 percent healthy. Eilene had included a note that she and Mike were so happy that they could hardly believe they were ever in danger of losing their marriage.

You can use the same miraculous metaphysical healing technique to cure your sick or dying marriage and to bring new health to the ailing marriages of any of your loved ones. Life and love are both wonderful gifts and you can use the miracle of metaphysical healing to keep them both one hundred percent healthy.

YOUR METAPHYSICAL HEALING TECHNIQUE FOR THE CURE OF A SICK OR DYING MARRIAGE

Follow these miraculous steps three times a day. You may use this failproof metaphysical healing method for yourself or for any of your loved ones simply by inserting their names in the appropriate places.

1. Select a location where you are not likely to be interrupted. Lie down or sit in a chair whose back is high enough to support your head.

2. Close your eyes and for a moment allow your consciousness to follow the intake and outflow of your breath without attempting to control it. Allow yourself to be completely aware of the new relaxation beginning to flood your mind and body.

3. Take a deep breath through your nostrils, extending your diaphragm as you inhale. Upon completion of inhalation completely relax your stomach muscles and allow your consciousness to follow the flow of breath through your body, bringing it to rest finally in the area of your head. Repeat this process three times and with each repetition become more and more aware of the total relaxation now filling your body and mind.

4. Repeat the following words to yourself mentally: "In the wisdom of my high self and through the power of my energized mind the miracle of metaphysical healing is now curing all sickness and injury in my marriage. I will that through the miracle of metaphysical healing my mate and I shall know a deeper and more satisfying love than we have ever known before. I release all grudges, resentments, feelings, and actions of any kind that are damaging to myself, my mate, or our marriage.

"Through the power of my energized mind and the miracle of metaphysical healing I will that love will be expressed in my marriage with ease and happiness. I further will that this love shall become more intense and more abundant with every passing day."

5. For a moment allow yourself to be completely aware of the intake and outflow of your breath without attempting to control it. Become totally aware of the complete relaxation now filling your body and mind.

6. Open your eyes and go about your daily life.

This miraculous technique of metaphysical healing cannot fail to cure the sick or dying marriage. It is yours to use today to bring complete health and total happiness to your own marriage or the marriage of any of your loved ones.

If you wish to use this miraculous technique to bring healing to the marriage of a friend or relative, simply insert their names in all appropriate places and carry out the step-by-step instructions as given above. You will find this miraculous technique of metaphysical healing for the sick and dying marriage 100 percent effective in all cases.

DRUG PROBLEMS CAN DESTROY FAMILY TIES— METAPHYSICAL HEALING CAN RESTORE THEM

Drug addiction is an illness prevalent in our society today which affects the lives of millions of individuals. Families have been torn apart through the sickness of their young people in developing an addiction to drugs. Most families are afraid or unequipped to deal with the drug problems of young people, and so communication within the family breaks down and family ties begin to die the slow death of a fatal sickness. Millions of dollars have been spent by local, state, and federal governments in an attempt to find a cure for drug addiction and the broken family ties that result from such addictions. In spite of all the money spent and all the man-hours expended, the traditional medical world has not yet discovered a way to cure drug addiction and restore the family ties ripped apart by this sickness. Despite the sincere efforts of many brilliant men in the health field, the best traditional medicine can offer to date is the substitution of one habit-forming drug for another. The methadone program is presented by traditional medicine as the lesser of two evils in the battle against drug addiction. Unlike the offerings of traditional medicine, the miracle of metaphysical healing offers a cure from drug addiction and a complete restoration of family ties that have been severed by that addiction.

PARENTS OF TEENAGE GIRL USE METAPHYSICAL HEALING TO CURE HER DRUG ADDICTION AND RESTORE HER RELATIONSHIP WITH HER FAMILY

Jeff and Sally K. were in sad shape when they came to see me for the first time. Their 15 year old daughter, Deborah, had slid from the habitual use of marijuana to an addiction to heroin. Jeff and Sally had learned of Deborah's addiction only four months prior to their visit to me, and during those four months they had taken Deborah to visit two physicians. Both doctors had suggested that Deborah be placed in the methadone program, but one important ingredient for such a placement was lacking. Deborah had no desire to give up her addiction to heroin.

The fact that Deborah's addiction to heroin had been discovered by her parents seemed to make Deborah more brazen in her use of this drug. She now demanded money from her parents in order to purchase the heroin she needed each day and threatened to steal or prostitute herself if her parents did not provide the money she needed.

"You can ask my wife, Deborah never acted like this before. She always loved her family and was taught that stealing and prostitution were very wrong.

"I know it's the drugs that are making her act the way she is and we want to help her get over them."

Pain was evident on the faces of both Deborah's parents as they talked about a daughter who was now all but lost to them.

"My husband is right. Deborah used to be such a sweet girl. Now it's as if she's not Deborah but somebody else. We want her back in the family and we want her cured of this drug thing.

"Jeff's brother told us about you and metaphysical healing and we figure maybe you could teach us to help Deborah. If there's anything that metaphysical healing can do to cure her of heroin and return her to us, we want to know about it.

"Please help us. We're willing to do anything to get our daughter back."

This same plea had echoed in the voices of many parents who had spoken with me in the past. Fathers and mothers seeking to reclaim their sons and daughters had sought out the miracle of metaphysical healing and had never once been disappointed in its results.

Jeff and Sally K. said they would follow the steps I had outlined for them in order to bring the miracle of metaphysical healing to their daughter, Deborah, cure her of heroin addiction, and return her to the family. Both said they would keep me posted on Deborah's progress.

Three months later my first update as to Deborah's progress came in the form of a visit from both her parents.

"We don't know how to thank you. Deborah is completely cured of her drug addiction, has gone back to school, and is home every evening. She's herself again and having our daughter back is too wonderful to put into words.''

"My wife speaks for me, too. We wanted our daughter back and we wanted her back badly. We're not educated people and we didr't know where else to turn for help until my brother mentioned you and metaphysical healing. At first I thought he was crazy to think that Sally and I could help Deborah when doctors couldn't help her. Well, I'm here to tell you that this miracle of metaphysical healing has taught us a lot about ourselves as well as giving us back our daughter. Sally and I know now that we can do a lot more than we ever thought we could in the past. This energized mind we all have is something else. I wish we had known about it when we were a lot younger, but I'll tell you one thing—now that we do know we're sure not going to waste it.

"We talked about what we could do to thank you for teaching us about metaphysical healing and Sally and I agreed that knowing that you're helping people must be a great comfort to you. God is letting you share in some of his work and there's nothing we could add to that except our thank you. We do thank you very much for teaching us how to get our daughter back in our family and get her over her sickness.''

Jeff K. called me six months later to tell me that Deborah was doing great and that the whole family was moving to another state where he and a brother were going to set up their own carpentry business. They were all looking forward to a very bright future.

YOUR MIRACLE TECHNIQUE OF METAPHYSICAL HEALING FOR THE CURE OF DRUG ADDICTION AND THE RESTORATION OF FAMILY TIES

Follow these failproof steps three times a day for yourself or for the family of a loved one. If you are performing this miracle exercise for another family, simply insert the names of these individuals in the appropriate places.

1. Select a location where you are not likely to be interrupted. Lie down or sit in a chair whose back is high enough to support your head.

2. Close your eyes and for a moment focus your consciousness on your intake and outflow of breath without attempting to

control it. Allow yourself to be completely aware of the new relaxation beginning to flow through your mind and body.

3. Take a deep breath through your nostrils, extending your diaphragm as you inhale. Upon completion of inhalation completely relax your stomach muscles and allow your consciousness to follow your breath, bringing it to rest finally in the area of your head. Repeat this process three times and with each repetition allow yourself to be more and more aware of the total relaxation now filling your body and mind.

4. Repeat the following words to yourself mentally: "In the wisdom of my high self and through the power of my energized mind and my ultra-mind I will that (here insert the name of the particular person to whom you are directing the miracle of metaphysical healing) be totally cured of the addiction to narcotics. I direct the unlimited power of my energized mind and my ultra-mind to the purpose of restoring this individual to perfect health and removing from this person all wishes, wants, and needs that are not in harmony with the balance of perfect health sought by the body and mind. The miracle of metaphysical healing is working now to bring the blessing of perfect health to this individual.

"With the same unlimited power of my energized mind and ultra-mind I further will that all family ties shall be restored to a condition of perfect health through the miracle of metaphysical healing. Perfect harmony and happiness shall live in this family through the miracle of metaphysical healing and the power of my energized mind and ultra-mind. Each family member shall attain a perfect harmony within himself and herself and shall live in complete balance and harmony with all other family members."

5. Take a deep breath through your nostrils, extending your diaphragm as you inhale. Upon completion of inhalation completely relax your stomach muscles and allow your consciousness to follow the breath, bringing it to rest finally in the area of the head. Repeat this process three times and with each repetition allow yourself to become more and more aware of the total and complete relaxation now filling your mind and body.

6. For a moment allow your consciousness to focus on the intake and outflow of your breath with no attempt to control it.

Give your consciousness once more to total awareness of the complete and harmonious relaxation now flooding your body and mind.

7. Open your eyes and go about your daily life.

This miraculous technique of metaphysical healing cannot fail to cure drug addiction and restore healthy family relationships. In a world plagued by drug addiction and the death of healthy family relationships this miraculous technique of metaphysical healing will allow you to restore perfect health and balance to your own family and to the families of those you love.

TEENAGERS CAN USE METAPHYSICAL HEALING TO RESTORE FAMILY RELATIONSHIPS

Many young people live in homes where the chief cause of family unhappiness can be traced to the behavior of the adults in that family. These young people can take full advantage of the unlimited power of energized mind in order to restore health and balance to their family situation.

Bill and Linda B. are two teenagers who used the miracle of metaphysical healing in order to restore happiness to a family torn apart through the alcoholic addiction of both parents and the subsequent lack of communication in the family resulting from that alcoholism. Bill and Linda asked my help in restoring happiness to their once harmonious home life.

At 15 and 16 years of age, Bill and Linda B. were already aware of the power of metaphysical healing. The help they needed now was the exact manner in which to use the miracle of metaphysical healing in order to cure their parents' alcoholism and restore happiness to their family relationships.

I explained to Bill and Linda that they were to use the metaphysical healing technique for alcoholism and add an additional paragraph to step number four. (You will find the metaphysical healing technique for alcoholism in Chapter four.)

Bill and Linda followed the metaphysical healing technique for alcoholism with the addition of a paragraph to be added to step number four, and in three months they notified me that their parents had stopped drinking. The family home life had become happy again and parents and teenagers were communicating mutual respect and love to each other.

Things have continued to get better in the B. home and according to Bill and Linda whom I hear from every three or four months, their parents have not touched a drop of alcohol in over two years.

You can use the same miraculous metaphysical healing technique for the cure of addiction to alcohol that restored happiness and health to the parents of Bill and Linda B. Simply follow the failproof method for the cure of alcoholism presented for you in Chapter four and add the following paragraph to step number four of this exercise.

MIRACLE PARAGRAPH TO BE ADDED TO STEP FOUR OF YOUR METAPHYSICAL HEALING TECHNIQUE FOR THE CURE OF ALCOHOLISM

"In the wisdom of my high self and through the power of my energized mind and my ultra-mind I will that all family relationships affected by the sickness of alcoholism will be restored to perfect health and balance. The miracle of metaphysical healing is working now to restore health and happiness in all family situations. Each family member will find new respect for himself or herself and will find and evidence the same respect and love for each other."

Don't suffer the pain of broken family relationships brought about by alcoholism any longer. Begin today to use this miracle technique that is guaranteed to cure alcoholic addiction and restore healthy and happy family relationships.

BROKEN FRIENDSHIPS CAN BE MORE PAINFUL THAN BROKEN BONES

Most of us can recall an event in our childhood where an argument or action separated us from a friend for a period of time. Children have a way of healing broken friendships very quickly and most likely if you can remember one such break in your childhood you can also remember a quick rekindling of that friendship. Oftentimes both friends apologized simultaneously or no apology was necessary on the part of either friend, but the friendship simply continued without reference to any break in the relationship. It is unfortunate that the majority of adults do not rekindle broken friendships as quickly or as easily as do children.

When arguments separate friends who are adults it is often hurt pride that stands in the way of the rekindling of the friendship. Often it is a matter of who will give in first and apologize and one adult tries to outlast the other in order that he or she will not be the first to say, "I'm sorry."

There are millions of adults in this world who suffer broken friendships today because of the holding of grudges and resentments by themselves or by their one-time friend.

The miracle of metaphysical healing offers to cure the broken friendship and restore a happy, balanced relationship between two friends quickly and without stepping on the pride of either individual. This miraculous healing method stands ready to help you today to rekindle old friendships that may have been lost to you in the past and to enjoy again the camaraderie of those who are lost to you through a break in the bonds of friendship.

METAPHYSICAL HEALING RESTORES A BROKEN FRIENDSHIP

It was Diane R. who sought my help in healing the bonds of friendship which had been broken between her and Paula W. for five months. Diane and Paula were both in their 30s and had been friends for 15 years. That friendship had ended with an argument that Diane could not even remember and since that time she had racked her brain in an attempt to understand what had actually happened to destroy her friendship with Paula W.

"I honestly don't know what the argument was about. I remember saying a lot of things I shouldn't have said and I remember Paula saying a lot of things that I know she wishes she hadn't said. I feel like an idiot for the whole thing, but every time I've tried to apologize to Paula she refuses to talk to me.

"We both have seven year old sons and the two of them play together every day. It's ridiculous that their mothers don't even speak after being friends for 15 years.

"I want you to teach me about the miracle of metaphysical healing so that I can restore my friendship with Paula. I've tried everything else and nothing has worked so far. I'd like you to teach me the method right away so I can start today. That silly argument has already wasted too much of our time."

Diane's attitude was certainly excellent and she listened intently as I explained the metaphysical healing technique she was to use in order to rekindle her friendship with Paula W. She said she would keep me informed on what happened and left looking and sounding very encouraged.

In less than a week Diane R. was on the phone to me and the warmth of her smile could be felt despite the physical distance between us.

"Talk about working fast! Paula called me the day before yesterday and said she wanted to talk with me. I met her for lunch and we both decided that whatever the argument was about it was silly to continue our broken friendship any longer.

"Last night my husband and I had dinner at Paula's home and everything is as if there was never a break in our friendship at all.

"Paula said she didn't know what possessed her to call me but that our friendship had been on her mind a lot during the last few days. You know, she couldn't remember what our argument was about, either.

"Thanks again for teaching me that metaphysical healing technique. I knew it would work but I never dreamed it would work so fast."

The miracle technique which restored Diane R.'s and Paula W.'s friendship is presented for you here. It cannot fail to bring metaphysical healing to broken friendships no matter what caused the break.

Friendship is a valuable gift. Don't waste another moment suffering the pain of a broken friendship when the miracle of metaphysical healing is waiting for you to use its miraculous power to rekindle broken relationships and enjoy lost friends once again.

YOUR MIRACULOUS FIRST AID KIT FOR BROKEN FRIENDSHIPS

Follow the steps in this miraculous exercise three times a day and it cannot fail to heal any broken friendship. You may also use this miracle technique to restore two loved ones who have parted friendship to a healthy and happy relationship again.

1. Select a location where you are not likely to be interrupted. Lie down or sit in a chair whose back is high enough to support your head.

2. Close your eyes and focus your attention on the intake and outflow of your breath with no attempt to control it. Allow

yourself to become aware of the new relaxation beginning to flood your mind and body.

3. Repeat the following words to yourself mentally: "In the wisdom of my high self and through the power of my energized mind and ultra-mind I will that the friendship between me and (here give the name of the person whose friendship you wish to regain; or insert both names of the two friends you are attempting to bring back together) be completely restored and that we shall stand in a position of mutual respect and love for each other. I direct all the power of metaphysical healing to the purpose of healing all resentments and grudges of any kind and replacing these destructive feelings with the positive feelings of love and mutual respect."

4. Take a deep breath through your nostrils, extending your diaphragm as you inhale. Upon completion of inhalation completely relax your stomach muscles and allow your consciousness to follow the breath, bringing it to rest finally in the area of your head. Repeat this process three times and with each repetition allow yourself to become more and more aware of the total relaxation now filling your body and mind.

5. Open your eyes and go about your daily life.

The miraculous technique for the restoration of friendship is now yours. It will allow you to restore all broken friendships and enjoy the blessings which friendship can bring into your life.

VITAMIN THOUGHTS—PREVENTIVE METAPHYSICAL HEALING THAT WILL SAVE YOU UNNECESSARY PAIN

By spending just ten minutes a day meditating on the following· thoughts you will add the strength of metaphysical healing to all your existing relationships. Simply recall these thoughts to mind and consider what they mean to you and to your relationships with other people.

1. All my fellow human beings and I are more alike than we are different.

2. I am a magnificent creation and through my interaction with other human beings I celebrate the beauty of all creation.

3. I am part of every human being and every human being is part of me.

4. Whenever two human beings interact they give spiritual growth to a new entity, a unique relationship that can exist only between the two of them. Each contributes his or her own uniqueness and the relationship that is born is a spiritual child of their creation.

5. Relationships are living things. They need care and love in order to grow and prosper.

6. It is in the give and take of relationships that human beings become truly human.

7. Each human being has something to teach you. Relate in order that you may learn and grow.

8. A beautiful mind, like a beautiful painting, was meant to be shared.

9. All things are relative and stand in relation to each other.

Give time to these vitamin thoughts every day in order that preventive metaphysical healing will keep your relationships happy and harmonious.

The miraculous techniques of metaphysical healing presented to you in this chapter will allow you to bring healing to any broken relationship. They are failproof miracle techniques and through their use you need never suffer the pain of a broken relationship again.

fifteen

Some Call Metaphysical Healing a Miracle

You have the power to work miracles. Through the power of metaphysical healing you can bring cures to diseases and injuries which traditional medicine considers virtually "incurable." With the power of your energized mind you can miraculously speed up the healing process so that injuries heal more quickly and sicknesses and diseases vanish in what would be considered an amazingly short time span.

A miracle may be defined as an event which fills people with wonder and amazement; it is an event which runs contrary to scientifically-accepted natural laws of the present. Through the unlimited power of your own energized mind you have the ability to bring miracles about in the field of healing. Through your knowledge of the miracle of metaphysical healing you are now a worker of wonders, a true miracle worker.

The unlimited power of your energized mind and your ultramind is at your disposal 24 hours a day. You are never more than a thought away from the ability to work a miracle in today's world. No one can take this knowledge from you and what person would be so foolish as to throw such knowledge away?

You are a different person from the individual who opened the cover of this book and began reading the first page. With each additional page and each additional chapter you read you gained new insights into yourself and into your own unlimited ability as a miracle worker. You learned the miraculous methods that would keep you in constant touch with the unlimited power within yourself and allow you to do what the majority of today's world considers impossible.

You have gained the knowledge to set aside diseases and injuries. You know the miraculous methods which will allow you to bring these miracles about.

In this book you have been able to share in the experiences of people just like yourself who discovered their own miraculous power to heal and changed their lives with the miracle of metaphysical healing. If this book were to contain all the individual cases where the miracle of metaphysical healing has brought perfect health to people stricken by disease and those afflicted with injuries, there would not be enough time in our world to read its contents. Because you have read this book your life can never again be the same. You now know the secrets for which human beings have searched for thousands of years. What you didn't know before you read this book could have hurt you a great deal. What you do know now that you have read this book will enable you to make disease, injury, sickness, and unhappiness only dim memories in your past. Through using the miraculous techniques you have learned your life from this point on will be filled with perfect harmony, health, and happiness.

If you have chosen to form or join a metaphysical healing group, you know that you have available to you at all times a metaphysical healing hot line. The combined unlimited power of a number of energized minds stands ready to help you at a moment's notice just as a metaphysical healing group once helped Cynthia W.

Cynthia W. had been a member of a healing group for one year. In an accident in her home, a window was shattered and the glass entered both of Cynthia's eyes. She was rushed to a hospital and doctors stated that Cynthia would be blind the rest of her life.

Cynthia's sister called one of the members of the metaphysical healing hot line and that member called another and so on until the entire metaphysical healing group was concentrating on sending the miracle of metaphysical healing to Cynthia W.'s eyes.

When the bandages were removed from Cynthia's eyes two days later, doctors were amazed by the fact that Cynthia could see clearly and that the wounds inflicted by broken glass were all but completely healed and were not leaving scar tissue. Two days later Cynthia W. was discharged from the hospital with 20/20 vision leaving behind an amazed medical staff who knew that by all rights Cynthia W. should be blind.

The miraculous power of energized mind directed through a metaphysical healing group had given Cynthia her eyesight when traditional medicine said that such a feat was an impossibility. Luckily for Cynthia and thousands of others like her, metaphysical healing groups do not have the word impossible in their vocabulary. You now possess the knowledge and ability to place the same kind of metaphysical healing hot line at your own disposal 24 hours a day.

The miracle power of your mind is your own best medicine in any situation. You can reach that miraculous power by a simple act of your will combined with the words, "I will to stand in the wisdom of my high self this very moment." In fact, using the miraculous techniques presented for you in this book you need never be out of contact with the unlimited power of your energized mind and your ultra-mind.

You have always been a natural born healer. With the knowledge and miraculous techniques presented to you in this book you are now able to tap your own unlimited power and use it to work the miracle of metaphysical healing in your everyday life.

You are truly a magnificent creation. You are a miracle worker!